GUIDE TO THE NEW MEDICINE

Guide to the NEW MEDICINE

What Works, What Doesn't

Hank Pizer

WILLIAM MORROW AND COMPANY, INC.
New York 1982

Library of Congress Cataloging in Publication Data

Pizer, Hank.
Guide to the new medicine.

Includes bibliographical references and index.
1. Therapeutic systems. 2. Quacks and quackery. I. Title.
R733.P59 1982 615.5 82-8233
ISBN 0-688-01314-7

Printed in the United States of America

First Edition

1 2 3 4 5 6 7 8 9 10

BOOK DESIGN BY JENNIE NICHOLS/LEVAVI & LEVAVI

To Chris and Katie

Acknowledgments

Special thanks to Alex Forman, licensed acupuncturist and physician assistant who coauthored the chapter on acupuncture. In addition, I would like to thank those healers who agreed to be interviewed for the book, and especially the creative and innovative staff of the Alternative Therapies Unit of San Francisco General Hospital. Finally, my sincerest appreciation goes to Elizabeth Frost Knappman at William Morrow who labored on the manuscript with me. Her efforts have enormously improved the quality of this work.

Contents

GUIDE TO THE NEW MEDICINE

c h a p t e r 1

Healers or Hucksters?

Americans have long thought they owed their good health and increased longevity to the health care provided by their physicians. Yet in the late 1960's they began to see this claim as propaganda from the ranks of organized medicine. Public health experts and consumers alike argued that conventional, allopathic medicine had become too impersonal, scientific, expensive, dangerous and narrow in its view of life.

This shift in perception helped to create a new health industry—an unregulated, multi-billion dollar business of acupuncturists, herbalists, faith healers, psychic surgeons, Rolfers, homeopaths, naturopaths and biofeedback practitioners. Not only did the new techniques grow, but older ones such as chiropractic, osteopathy and herbalism—on the fringe for many years—also increased in popularity. Many physicians who had been trained in conventional medical practices also chose to practice "holistically," or to take up homeopathy, acupuncture, hypnosis, orthomolecular medicine, relaxation or some other new technique.

Like all new industries, the alternative healers use largely unproven methods. Many of their practices will eventually change or be proven worthless or will become incorporated into conventional medicine. While this is no different from allopathic Western medicine (where treatments change every few years), it should be a lesson to both consumer and practitioner to be wary of healing "fads" and unproven practices.

Alternative healers have been somewhat reluctant to look at their own work in an objective manner. Many are openly critical of the scientific method, and have rejected experimentation as a means of justifying their work. In addition, the newness of the industry and its shortage of research money and institutions have made it difficult to prove its methods.

But for the consumer, this is a trying and dangerous situation. Where do you find a reputable healer? Which therapy should you choose? If you suffer from high blood pressure, should you try relaxation, biofeedback, acupuncture, hypnosis or exercise? Should you try more than one method at once? While these questions come up when one sees a traditional physician, in alternative healing there is even more uncertainty. Moreover, in illness there is always the potential for creating harm when an important diagnosis is missed or the wrong treatment is applied.

In this book we will evaluate the efficacy of each of the new therapies and offer guidelines for choosing and evaluating your own medical care. But remember, good standards do not exist, and each client must approach the new healers with a critical eye.

The Growth of Alternative Healing

The alternative healing industry is composed of an array of healers. Some claim to be "holistic" in that they treat the entire person; others provide specialized care with specific techniques. Both kinds have undergone a rapid growth in the last decade.

For instance, in 1970 there were 13,729 chiropractors in the United States. By 1980 they numbered 20,000. In 1980 their average income was more that $65,000. (More than half of all chiropractors make over $83,000.) And there are more than 8½ million *new* patients seeing chiropractors every year.

Holism has also grown enormously. The American Holistic Medical Association, a group of physicians who practice holistic medicine, had only 220 members at their founding meeting in 1978. In the first year they doubled their membership. Dr. Elmer Cranton, President of AHMA, estimates that there are now over 2,000 holistic *physicians* throughout the country, and that:

> [T]here are another 10,000 to 20,000 closet progressives, who know the present system is faulty, but who aren't up to "challenging the establishment."

Dr. Cranton estimates that 10 times as many patients are seeking out holistic doctors for care as 10 years ago. These numbers include only medical doctors practicing "holistically"; certainly there are more patients seeking care from nonphysicians who call themselves holists.

Similar growth has taken place in other areas. The American Biofeedback Society has grown from 12 members in 1970 to over 2,000 in 1980. During the same period, homeopathy has increased from a handful of practitioners to more than 600. When James Reston reported in 1972 that the Chinese used acupuncture for postoperative nausea, few people had even heard of the practice. Since that time thousands of new patients seek out this treatment each year. The New England School of Acupuncture started in 1976 in Massachusetts as the first such school in the country. Since then it has quadrupled its student population. Among other practices that did not exist 10 years ago are Rolfing, Feldenkrais, reflexology, polarity, the Bates Method, Benjamin Massage, Iridology and negative ionization. Today, these practices are chic for the middle class and wealthy.

Is It Just Faith?

Healers have always held prominent positions in society. Although almost all of their remedies would be considered useless today, the doctors of the past successfully treated most of the ills of their time. Leeches, lizard's blood, crocodile dung, the teeth of swine, putrid meat, fly specs, bezoar stones could all effectively heal the sick. For instance, in the late eighteenth century an English medical paper described a cure for a toothache that worked 75% of the time. It advised the patient to "fill his mouth with milk and shake it until it became butter."

The record of allopathic medicine in claiming cures

with nonspecific and sometimes harmful treatments continues into the modern era. Treatments for *angina pectoris* have included taking heart muscle extracts, hormones, cobra venom, anticoagulants, vitamins, and tranquilizers; and enduring treatments from X rays to the interruption of the internal mammary artery in the chest, or the scraping of the epidardium (the outer layer of the heart). Moreover, papers have been published in reputable journals that have touted the effectiveness of these methods for improving or eliminating chest pain. Yet today, none of these treatments is considered beneficial for angina.

It is extremely difficult to accurately evaluate how well any kind of medical treatment works. At first studies are published by "enthusiasts" who claim fantastic results in 70 to 90% of cases. Later, "skeptics" repeat these studies and find the treatments to be valueless. In the end any therapy may be effective in one-third of cases. This 30% effectiveness is due to the "placebo effect," in which the human body heals itself by harnessing its own mental, spiritual and physical resources.

Dr. Kenneth Pelletier, Assistant Clinical Professor in the Department of Psychiatry at the University of California School of Medicine in San Francisco, puts it this way:

> Every therapy works for someone, somewhere, some of the time. There isn't a single therapeutic intervention that I can think of that doesn't have someone who has been helped by it. So there is an element of hit and miss involved that may never be reduceable. . . .

For instance, take the example given above of the surgical procedure once used to treat angina, where the surgeon tied closed the internal mammary artery in the chest.

Enthusiastic physicians reported that over 35% of the patients treated had complete relief of their chest pain, and that 75% had improvement in their symptoms. However, when the operation was repeated by "skeptical" surgeons who opened the chest but did not tie off the artery, similar results were obtained. The patients, believing that the surgery was going to help them, reported feeling better.

Furthermore, when the surgery was repeated by physicians who conveyed doubt to the patients, less than 10% had improvement in their chest pain. So it often is the attitude of the healer, not the healer's technique or expertise, that results in a cure. We feel better because of our *faith* in the healer and the healing environment.

Even more dramatic is this story of a cancer patient.

> [In this patient tumors] the size of oranges were present in the neck, axilla [arm pits] and groin, chest and abdomen. The spleen and liver were greatly enlarged. The patient was resistant to all treatment, was completely bedridden, and his life-expectancy was thought to be a matter of days or weeks. Despite this, the patient was not without hope because he had heard of the favorable publicity with which the newspapers had reported a new anticancer drug called Krebiozen. The patient learned that the drug was to be tried at the hospital at which he was confined. His entreaties for the drug were finally granted, although with reluctance and pessimism.
>
> The patient's response was astonishing. After one day of treatment, the tumor masses melted to half their original size. Within 10 days all signs of his disease vanished. He breathed normally and was discharged. After two months of almost perfect health, conflicting and pessimistic reports about Krebiozen began to appear in the newspapers. The

> patient lost hope and relapsed to his original state. The physician, however, rekindled the patient's hope by telling him not to believe what he read, that the drug deteriorated with standing, and that a new super-refined, double-strength drug was to arrive the following day. The patient was then given water injections and his optimistic expectations were restored. Recovery was even more dramatic than before. He became ambulatory and was discharged, and continued symptom-free for over two months. The remission continued until a few days after the press published an American Medical Association announcement that nationwide tests showed Krebiozen to be a worthless drug in the treatment of cancer. Within a few days the patient was readmitted to the hospital and succumbed in less than 48 hours. (Lief, 1963)

The placebo effect also plays a role in alternative medicine. By extending warmth, empathy and understanding to their patients, the new healers may harness the placebo effect more effectively than conventional healers. This does not imply dishonesty on the part of the alternative therapists, but raises the question of the validity of the specific new techniques that they employ.

Leonard Duhl is a psychiatrist and professor at the School of Public Health at the University of California at Berkeley. He has been both personally and professionally part of the alternative medicine movement for many years. He explained to me how the new healers harness the placebo effect:

> Medical care has been more geared towards the care of the seriously ill, and not towards the kvetches of ordinary daily life. The medical system is not set up to deal with the simple problems of "I hurt." . . .

> You find that doctors don't really touch [their patients while] alternative healers are really putting hands on. Also in medicine there is a tendency to have the physician up high and the client down low. In alternative care healers act as co-equals. They call their patients "clients," and share their experiences.

The question then arises, "Should people pay money and put faith in these alternative practices, or can they find other ways to heal themselves?"

The Politics of the New Healers

The new healers ask to be judged on their own merits, not according to the standards of conventional Western medicine. Yet much of the interest in the new healers is a political and social expression of dislike and distrust for industrial America and allopathic medicine. The growth of these healers came during the late 1960's and early 1970's, when great cultural changes were sweeping the nation. Pamela Picker of the Berkeley Holistic Health Center described this to me: "A whole set of new diseases has developed. Holistic [medicine] addresses the bottom-line issues of survival. . . . You hear about surviving in the 80's. I think that this is a lot of what holistic [medicine] is addressing at this point. It is the insurance of getting through this difficult transition in time."

Many turned to the new medicine in the 1960's and 70's as a way of forging a new social direction. The new healers developed out of the human potential movement, the women's movement, an interest in Eastern philosophy and in the environment. Their popularity also came about as the result of criticism about national health policies that was not answered by conventional medicine.

Medical practitioners realize today that the health-care system is not a particularly good way to change society, and probably not all that powerful a means for changing individuals. Medicine in fact is notoriously apolitical in its outlook—except for issues that relate directly to the incomes of its practitioners. The criticisms that the new healers level at the society do not go beyond the narrow limitations of health care, and these focus on changing the individual and not the society. For instance, Michael Jansen, a physician who practices orthomolecular medicine at the New England Health Foundation in Cambridge, Massachusetts, explained it to me this way: "Society consists of individuals and if those individuals do not change . . . you can't change the society that is composed of them. You can't expect to get responsible leaders from an irresponsible public."

Health-care providers regard their work much like "Christian good deeds" and disdain working together on common problems or large social goals, outside of the care of their individual patients. Therefore the new healers probably will not have a profound effect on changing American society or the medical system.

Healers or Hucksters?

Any new, rapidly growing and unregulated industry will inevitably contain a broad range of people. Some will be effective, honest and make advances in their profession; others will merely profit from the tide of events. Unfortunately, in medicine a patient can lose more than just money in the search for cures. This is especially true if untrained, unscrupulous or capricious practitioners are allowed to give health care.

Dr. Jerome Schofferman at the Alternative Therapies Unit of San Francisco General Hospital says: "There has been such a proliferation of individuals who have been able to call themselves healers, without background or credentials, without any need to document their abilities, that some clients have obviously suffered through neglect or mistakes."

There are few standards for the bulk of the alternative healing methods. Licensing exams, standardized curriculums, registration by the states or professional societies, standards of practice and procedures for reviewing incompetent or impaired practitioners are rare. Some people take a seminar for a weekend or two and claim to be healers.

Some sort of accountability must take place. Regulation should not necessarily be by the conventional medical establishment, which has been opposed to new healing disciplines. Yet the new healers need to standardize their professions and create some order out of the heterogenous group of nonphysician practitioners that now practices alternative healing methods. Not only will this help protect the public, but it will forward the alternative healing industry.

The Next Step—Consumer's Choice

The future of the new healers in America will depend on their ability to prove their effectiveness. Over the last 30 years the cost of health care in the United States has skyrocketed from $12 billion (4.5% of the Gross National Product in 1950) to over $250 billion (about 10% of the GNP) in 1980. At the same time there has been no change in the death rate, and life expectancy in the United States lags behind that of Sweden, France, Netherlands, Canada, England and Wales. If the goal is improved health, society should be willing to find new ways for attaining it. Placing the bulk of health-care dollars into the hands of conventional medicine is not likely to help us realize this goal.

At the same time the alternative healers have to demonstrate that they stand for more than a criticism of allopathic medicine or the activation of the placebo effect. As Dr. Richard Svihus wrote:

> Most alternative therapies, which may not have been proved effective by scientific methods, must depend in part or entirely on faith for their effectiveness. Faith can be an effective part of the healing process, and probably is the cause of many spontaneous remissions of presumably incurable diseases. But the danger inherent in alternative therapies is that one may come to believe that the therapies are effective in and of themselves, without taking into account the component of faith. Licensure of alternative practitioners could result in institutionalizing techniques which are therapeutic only when carried out by certain persons who are capable of generating faith on the part of others. (Svihus, 1977)

The origins of Western medicine, traditional Oriental medicine and the tribal medicine of virtually all peoples demonstrate the validity of treating the mind and body with a variety of techniques. Unfortunately we have strayed from that tradition. As medicine has progressed in the scientific direction, this philosophy has been put aside for an emphasis on the body as a set of chemical reactions that take place on the cellular level. As we shall see in

Chapter 2, this has been a basic criticism asserted by alternative medicine. The future may bring a synthesis of these two approaches and better guidelines for the client who needs medical care. But whatever the future, resting an entire healing system on the beliefs of client and practitioner is clearly not enough.

c h a p t e r 2

The Origins of the Alternative Healers

American allopathic medicine is a powerful system that resists criticism and competition. If consumers felt that it was adequately meeting their needs, it would be difficult for the new medicine to gain a foothold. After all, we are brought into the world by doctors, raised in part by our pediatricians and seen in our moments of need by our internists. Straying from this system is a willful break with our earliest memories and associations.

At the heart of our search for new treatments is the debate between medicine as *science* and medicine as *art.* Traditional medicine has shut out the individual—human, empathetic and artistic—in favor of the technology and science of healing. The new healers represent a reaction to this technological trend, and place a renewed emphasis on the traditions of family, creativity and the human spirit.

The emphasis on science and technology in medicine begins in the way we choose students for medical training. Medical colleges select students who do well in the basic sciences, not those who flourish in the arts and humanities. Doctors-to-be spend their adolescence studying science, competing for grades and looking at the technology of the world. They learn to reduce life to equations in the chemistry laboratory or specimens under the microscope. By shutting out history, art, politics and culture from the academic background of medical students, admissions committees take in the narrowest of students. The extreme competitiveness of admission to medical school forces young people to go into the basic sciences from early adolescence, and this perspective continues into their clinical practice of medicine.

This emphasis, of course, continues into medical training. The few courses that are taught about ethics, the family or human interaction are the "gut" courses—the easy ones that provide a break from the grueling pattern of memorizing enormous amounts of scientific information for endless examinations in anatomy, chemistry, pharmacology and medicine.

The testing method in medical training further enhances this impersonal mentality. While in other fields—history, law, or education—students write out essays that explain a point of view, in medicine examinations are by multiple-choice, and are corrected by machines. Those students who get through most easily are the ones who become facile at memorizing and reciting facts.

Dr. Robert Mendelsohn, associate professor of preventive medicine and community health at the University of Illinois, says:

> The admissions tests and policies of medical schools virtually guarantee that the students who get in will make poor doctors. The quantitative tests, the Medical College Admissions Test, and the reliance on grade-point averages funnel through a certain type of personality who is unable and unwilling to communicate with people. (Mendelsohn, R., 1980)

At medical schools the science and technology of healing have suppressed all else. At Albany Medical Center, the following procedure is taught as the correct method of taking a family history:

> State health, or cause of death of parents, siblings; with age at time of death. Inquire specifically regarding tuberculosis, rheumatism, diabetes, cancer, heart and kidney disease, nervousness or insanity. Asthma, hay fever, migraine, hypertension, obesity, bleeding tendency. If there is reason, as in the case of tuberculosis, obtain history of grandparents, uncles, aunts or other persons living in the household. (Medical History and Physical Examination, Albany Medical College, 1973)

Students are taught to focus on medical pathology. The intellectual rewards go to this student who finds the obscure disease. As Dr. Samuel Shem (the pen name for a Boston area physician) says in his medical satire, *House of God,* when a doctor hears hoofbeats, "he looks for a zebra."

This kind of outlook does not teach students to consider the quality of human life—the love, security, and sense of responsibility that eventually become important indicators of individual health.

Alternative Healing Emerges

Alternative healers argue that allopathic medicine has lost the human perspective. They point out that it encourages expensive, often dangerous procedures instead of promoting the personal and social health needed to prevent disease. They point to the fact that in the 1970's over 70% of physicians were specialists; that although there was a doctor for every 645 people (a reasonable ratio), there was only one family physician or GP for every 4,771 people (an unreasonable figure). We had invested billions into treating the common aches and pains of living with expensive tests, drugs and surgery.

The new healers have therefore tried to replace technology with warmth, understanding and empathy. If the average doctor visit took 10 minutes, then the new healers would spend at least an hour with a patient. If the conventional doctor touched patients only with a stethoscope, then the new healers would make a point to have physical contact with their clients. If regular doctors gave out millions of useless and sometimes dangerous prescriptions, the new healers would emphasize diet, exercise, stress reduction, more fulfilling lifestyles and herbs. If technology and specialization were destroying the healing relationship, then the new methods would emphasize caring over curing.

Dr. Richard Ingrasci is a holistically oriented physician who trained at Cornell and Harvard and the Health Director of Interface, a Boston area holistic educational association. Echoing how far medicine has strayed from what human beings really need in the healing setting, he says that: "If you go to the greatest medical institutions in our culture, the Massachusetts General Hospital, Beth Israel Hospital, Harvard Medical School, you will notice something very striking. No attention at all has been paid to the quality of the environment. It's a machine, it's cold, it's computers all over the place. People walk by very fast not paying attention to each other. You pay a price for that ambiance in terms of the eventual outcome [of the patient care]."

From Plato to Koch

How did this emphasis on the science and technology of healing come about? From the time of Plato until the twentieth century, physicians had to practice holistically. This meant taking into account the social and spiritual state of the patient as well as analyzing the condition of the body. In reality they had little choice, since their knowledge of the biology and pathology of the body was extremely limited, and there were few medical treatments that worked for specific diseases. Doctors relied on their personal magnetism and on *faith.* They conveyed to the patient a belief that they could help, and in turn the patient believed that they would.

By the late nineteenth century this system of healing began to change. The scientific method had already produced major advances in physics and chemistry that had been successfully applied to the chemical industry, steel making, the production of munitions, transportation and manufacture of all sorts. We had entered the scientific revolution that completed the industrial revolution of the prior 150 years.

Medicine and biology were slower than chemistry,

physics and engineering in incorporating the scientific method. To begin with, it was more difficult to understand the intricacies of the cell and its biochemical operations than to design experiments in physics and inorganic chemistry. Not until some important discoveries were made in using the microscope and dyes to stain for microbes, along with laboratory techniques for culturing bacteria, did medical science take a great leap forward.

The initial breakthroughs were made by bacteriologists who discovered that infections were caused by microscopic organisms and not by the "vapors" and "miasmas" that had been thought to be responsible for the epidemics and plagues of human history. Until recently, infections were our principal killers: diphtheria, cholera, malaria, smallpox, typhus, tuberculosis and pneumonia. Thus the bacteriologists' illumination of the causes of these illnesses was the medical breakthrough that altered our prior history.

The German physician Robert Koch (1843–1910) was a model for the doctor as scientist. While traveling through Germany in performing his duties, he spent his spare time working with the microscope he carried with him. In 1876 he made his first major discovery by studying the complete life cycle of the anthrax bacteria, which produces a serious infection in man and animals. By careful analysis Koch demonstrated that the tiny organism he raised in a pure culture could be inoculated into an animal and produce disease.

By doing this Koch proved that diseases had a specific cause that could be identified; illness was no longer the will of God or bad luck. Science—at least in the rationalist perspective—had found the answer to human ills. Koch soon became very famous for this work, traveling throughout the world to study infectious disease. He culminated an illustrious career with the discovery of the tuberculosis bacterium.

Today, Koch's *postulates* stand as a model for the application of scientific principles to medical research. These state that a cause-and-effect relationship must be established between a disease and an agent producing the disease. In effect, Koch's legacy was the "one-cause, one-disease" mentality; and although his postulates were meant to apply to infectious diseases, their ideology eventually became applied to all of medicine. His work was a milestone in the advancement of the philosophy of allopathic medical science.

Although simplistic in its philosophy, the cause-and-effect relationship between agents and events and their ultimate production of disease continues as our principal reductionistic (logical) thought process. This is important to remember because later, when we look at homeopathy, we will see a direct challenge to this scientific perspective.

Meanwhile the effect of the bacteriologists' discoveries was to silence the social critics, reformers and revolutionaries who sought to push medicine into the political arena. The nineteenth century was a time of great social unrest in Europe. The industrialization of society had brought massive social upheaval and the ills of the modern city. Pollution, inadequate sewage disposal, impure drinking water, lack of refrigeration and most of all appalling factory conditions created extreme health hazards. Like the holists and environmentalists of today, the social critics of the past century sought to use the medical system to speak out against these evils.

But the discoveries of the bacteriologists permitted medicine to use science to stay out of the political forum.

It was easier and more appealing for both physicians and governments to view disease as created by impersonal microorganisms than to see the industrial system as the culprit. And though the bacteriologists quickly discovered the link between unsanitary conditions and the spread of infectious diseases, it was still possible to focus on the spread of pathogens rather than on the underlying social context. Today we now know that the control of tuberculosis, dysentery, and many other serious infections has been largely due to sanitation, nutrition and other public health measures. Medical treatment has been only a minor factor in this improvement.

Relying solely on a biomedical perspective is now considered a narrow and conservative view. Today most public health experts readily accept the criticisms of the new healers and social critics of the nineteenth century, who linked lifestyle, environment and occupation with illness. Moreover, with the elimination of infectious disease as a primary killer, Western medical scientists have had to move beyond the "one-cause, one-disease" mentality. Heart disease, stroke and cancer clearly have multiple underlying causes, as do accidents, suicides and homicides—the fourth, ninth and eleventh most significant killers.

The feelings of the new healers may be summarized by Dr. William McGarey in the *Journal of Holistic Medicine* (Volume 1, 1976): "In the field of organized medicine, historically we found man affected with disease; so we became very much interested in destroying the disease process. . . . So we scientific individuals became interested in the disease, and we got away from the human being."

Perhaps the last gasp in the "one-cause, one-disease" model occurred in the early 1970's when the Nixon administration went to "war" to find a viral cause for cancer. Despite billions invested in this theory, the notion currently promoted by the epidemiologists, environmentalists and alternative healers is that 60 to 90% of cancers are caused by lifestyle, occupation and environment. Dr. John Knowles, past president of the Rockefeller Foundation and one-time chief at the Memorial Sloan-Kettering Cancer Center in New York, summed up this view:

> . . . over 99% of us are born healthy and made sick as a result of personal misbehavior and environmental conditions. . . . Alas the medical profession isn't interested because the intellectual, emotional and financial rewards of the present system are too great and because there is no incentive and very little demand for change. (Knowles, 1975)

As we shall see, there is a growing demand for this system to make enormous changes.

Origins of Holistic Medicine

As stated earlier, holistic medicine gained favor in the 1970's in opposition to the sterile, scientific laboratory medicine of the modern era. Its proponents were often graduates of the highly touted, research-oriented medical colleges. Not only did they take direct objection to the heritage of Koch's postulates, but they pointed out that this approach treated disease only after it had struck.

Interestingly, the origins of the word holistic have nothing to do with medicine. It was coined by Jan Smuts, a military man who became Prime Minister of South Africa. In 1926 he wrote a book entitled *Holism and Evolution* in which he held that individual organisms and social systems were entities greater than the sum of their individual parts. He saw in the evolution of species and societies growth until the whole is complete. In biological terms this means that organisms can continue to develop to a fullness of potential. Holism allows for a spiritual view of human life that conventional scientific medicine either ignores or represses.

By adopting holism, *avant-garde* healers can broaden their horizons and get away from the deadly, stifling approach to human beings as pathological processes. At the same time, holism permits physicians to focus on wellness as well as illness. A concept of *high-level wellness* arose which incorporated the ideas that Abraham Maslow and the self-actualization movement in psychology had been espousing. George Leonard, formerly senior editor at *Look* magazine and a proponent of the new medicine, described this new philosophy:

> Psychology entered a new era when Abraham Maslow began studying people who are at their peak mentally and emotionally, rather than pathological individuals who had always preoccupied that science. In the same way medicine is transformed when it begins looking at above-average physical fitness, extraordinary alertness, and awareness, and the tingling sense of well-being that affords high resistance to disease. (Leonard, 1976)

Holism also drew from other political and cultural movements that began in the 1960's. Americans had developed an interest in Oriental culture in the 1950's, and expanded it during the drug revolution of the mid-1960's. Oriental medicine and acupuncture had a naturally holistic approach, combining a philosophy of opposites (the Yin and Yang symbols in traditional Chinese cosmology), and an emphasis on natural healing with acupressure and herbs. Moreover, Oriental medicine was based on ancient traditions that predated the scientific era of Koch and the bacteriologists. Empirically, it seemed to work and, like homeopathy, was based on observation rather than laboratory manipulation. It included the concept that there was a life force, or spirit, that would be healthy when the organism was healthy, and sick when the inner spirit was ill.

Holistic medicine also drew support from the environmentalists, who amassed enormous amounts of evidence that American industry, the automobile and the materialistic culture of the post-World War II era were destroying American society. The women's movement gave a direct challenge to conventional medicine, which had a notorious tradition of sexism, elitism and the exclusion of women, and an untoward propensity for medical intervention in treating women. The movement effectively pointed out the excesses of radical mastectomy, the abuse of estrogen replacement after menopause, and the pattern of unnecessary hysterectomies and cesarian deliveries.

In the women's self-help movement in health care, women encouraged each other to examine themselves, to seek other women for health care and to learn about their own bodies. Holism also encouraged responsibility for one's own health, and both points of view were naturally supportive. Women sought natural childbirth, midwifery, less invasive medical procedures (feeling there were too many hysterectomies and cesarian births) and self-examination of the breast and vagina, and fought the objections of the obstetricians and gynecologists. While the conventional medical establishment had conducted a vitriolic attack on midwifery beginning with the turn of this century, midwives all over the country began to thrive, and in some places claimed to have better results than conventionally trained obstetricians. Thus, holistic medicine is the result of the failure of science and materialism to make us happy, and of the drive for equality among various groups in American society against whom traditional medicine has discriminated.

Chiropractic in America

Unlike holistic medicine, chiropractic grew out of the lay-healing traditions in America. Its founder, Daniel David Palmer (1845–1913), was a traveling merchant who for reasons that remain unclear began lay-healing in a factory loft in Burlington, Iowa in 1886. For 10 years his reputation grew by word of mouth, and on September 18, 1895, he began the chiropractic profession by performing the first spinal adjustment.

He did this for a janitor named Harvey Lillard, who miraculously seemed to be cured of his hearing loss as a result of an adjustment of the neck. In Palmer's words:

> I replaced the displaced fourth dorsal vertebrae by one move, which restored his hearing fully. (Haldeman, 1979)

It is not surprising that an unconventional profession like chiropractic would begin in this unusual fashion. Both D.D. Palmer and his son, Bartlett Joshua Palmer, were unusual people. Both were charismatic, critical of the conventional medical establishment, and approached chiropractic with the zeal of a great promoter. B. J. Palmer has been described as the P.T. Barnum of medicine—a man who traveled throughout the country spreading the word of chiropractic.

By 1896, D.D. Palmer had opened up a small school for teaching spinal manipulation, the "Dr. Palmer's School and Cure." The art of chiropractic was still virtually unknown to the public. By 1902 only 15 students had graduated from the school, but in that very special year, B.J. Palmer began to take on the role of leader of the movement. And from then until B.J.'s death in 1961, he remained a reigning figure in the profession.

B.J. Palmer looked the part of lay-healer. He sported white suits and wore his black hair down to his shoulders. From his first moments in chiropractic he launched into a flamboyant and continual attack on allopathy. At every turn he proselytized chiropractic, claiming that it could cure all illness, treat the insane and even deliver babies.

B.J. also put together the largest museum of human spines of his day, and encouraged the early use of X rays for diagnosis. In 1924 he began to tout a new medical device —the neurocalometer—that sensed heat changes in the body. These temperature changes were supposed to indicate the presence of subluxed (slipped) vertebrae, which then could be manipulated by the chiropractor. (Eventually this proved to be a useless device.) In 1935, B.J. pioneered a largely useless instrument for reading brain waves. Throughout his years as leader of the profession, he encouraged chiropractic to open schools, hospitals and clinics, and to take on the most difficult cases that had not been aided by allopathic medicine.

After B.J. Palmer took over the leadership of chiropractic from his father, D.D. left Davenport, Iowa, to spread the word of the new profession. Finally, he went to the Indian Territory, Canada, Oregon and California. While in Los Angeles to attend the graduation ceremony of the chiropractic school, and walking in the school parade, he was struck by a car driven by his son B.J. He died three months later, amidst rumors of patricide. (Haldeman, 1979)

The history of chiropractic demonstrates the zeal with which new healers must work to survive in the face of allopathic hostility. From its early beginnings, chiropractic met an intense legal and professional opposition from organized medicine. In 1906 D.D. Palmer was jailed in Scott County, Iowa for practicing medicine without a license. A witch hunt against chiropractors continued throughout the country through the 1950's. In 1949 the proceedings of the New York State Medical Society declared:

> . . . we are not talking about the licensing of chiropractors . . . we are talking about the destruction of chiropractors . . . the elimination of murderers. (Haldeman, 1979)

In 1921, 450 of the approximately 600 chiropractors in the state of California were tried for practicing medicine without a license and went to jail rather than pay a fine. In the next year 100 were jailed in New York State.

Yet chiropractic survived, largely because of the commitment and faith of its practitioners. Chiropractors saw their profession in a religious fashion—believing that their persecution at the hands of allopathy indicated the worthiness of their profession. In 1915 Howard Nutting wrote in the journal *The Chiropractor:*

> . . . keep bravely on until the flag of chiropractic is unfurled in every town and hamlet: on until every asylum for the insane, for the inebriate, and for the feeble-minded shall be without occupants, or until the penitentiaries and reformatories are deserted and their crumbling walls and rusted bolts stand only as silent testimonials to the success of chiropractic. (Haldeman, 1975)

From the first, chiropractors said they could cure every disease, because they thought all maladies were due to the subluxation of the spinal bones. Today even the most zealous chiropractors would be embarrassed by such claims, but given the extraordinary abuse their profession has had from the medical establishment, it is understandable that their claims had to be grandiose.

Today, doctors of chiropractic claim that 74% receive referrals from M.D.'s. Moreover, with an average income of over $65,000, chiropractors can now socially rub shoulders with physicians. The economics of medicine are extremely important; now that chiropractic has made it economically into the mainstream of healing, allopathy is less critical of its lay traditions.

The survival of chiropractic also stands as a blow to the concept of medicine as a science, rather than an art. Unlike the bacteriologists of the nineteenth and early twentieth centuries, chiropractic was not based on laboratory investigation. From the very beginning it was an empirical profession, whose principals had no medical or scientific training. But while the science of chiropractic has improved over the years, its first patients obviously were not frightened off by the lack of credentials of its practitioners. Patients took it on faith that chiropractors had learned something about health and the human body. To some extent they must have also accepted the great claims of the new healing practice. All of this stands directly in opposition to every tenet of allopathic medicine.

Homeopathy

Homeopathy is a third major force in alternative healing. While holism grew out of allopathy, criticizing its cold, narrow, laboratory perspective, and chiropractic out of lay-healing, homeopathy developed with a different *scientific* perspective.

Modern homeopathy began with Samuel Hahnemann (1755–1843), a German physician who saw illness as an expression of disorder within the vital force *(elan vital)* of the body. Rather than seeking remedies that would suppress symptoms such as pain or fever, Hahnemann considered these signs to be positive expressions of the body's innate healing capability.

Hahnemann began with an entirely different scientific method of investigation. While traditional allopathy studied individuals with diseases, Hahnemann studied normal people. He actually began with himself, by ingesting doses of quinine. He noted that the quinine produced symptoms similar to those of the malaria that it was useful for treating. From this he developed the notion that *like cured like,* or the *Law of Similars,* as it has come to be called.

Harris Coulter, a medical historian, has outlined the alternative philosophical direction that Hahnemann created.

> Interpreting the patient's symptoms as positive signs of reaction, Hahnemann logically concluded that the cure would be brought about by any drug or medicinal substance which supported this reaction, and it was this which led him to the idea of cure through similars. The medicine which, in a healthy person, gives rise to precisely the symptom-pattern of the given patient is the medicine which will cure that patient. (Coulter, 1977)

Thus, Hahnemann developed a descriptive or empirical approach to scientific inquiry. His study involved giving hundreds of plant and mineral substances to normal people and observing their responses. Unlike modern medical science, Hahnemann did not strive to understand the underlying process of healing, but accepted that the body had a natural ability to correct itself in response to stress. This act of giving a substance and observing the symptoms that resulted was called a *proving,* and it is striking in its difference from what we today would consider to be proof.

Next, Hahnemann realized that it was the *smallest* amount of a remedy that produced the most beneficial effects. Contrary to the medical notion of his time and ours —where large doses of drugs are often used—homeopathy developed the concept of *potentizing* substances by diluting them. Homeopathic remedies are in fact so diluted that they may have no chemical evidence of the healing substance in the solution that is taken by the patient. In other words, to the homeopath—less means more. Not only does this represent a challenge to the drug industry, but it leads to a different scientific concept of the molecular basis of the cell and its response to chemicals. As one can imagine, homeopathic remedies have been criticized as placebos since the very beginning.

An appeal of homeopathy and of giving very small doses of remedies is that it is extremely safe. In an age in which allopathic medicine has been criticized for its extreme interventions, homeopathy represents a conservative approach to healing. Homeopathy also makes a different fundamental distinction between the symptoms, the patient and the illness. Each individual's symptoms are a unique expression of the disorder in his or her life force or vital energy. As Dr. James Stephenson of New York points out:

> He [Hahnemann] did not regard the patient's signs and symptoms as necessarily bad and therefore to be removed. Instead, Hahnemann believed that these signs and symptoms represented an attempt by the body to heal itself. According

> to this view, the signs and symptoms do not represent the *illness,* but the *reaction* of the person to his illness. The illness and the reaction to the illness are separate. (Stephenson, 1960)

These distinctions fit in well with our contemporary criticism of medicine as solely interested in organs, tissues, and parts of the body rather than the whole person.

Finally, homeopathy stands as a criticism and alternative to the existing reductionistic science of allopathy. While other alternative healing methods have avoided or have been unable to establish a total perspective and underlying foundation for their healing, homeopathy has developed one.

This is particularly important in respect to the question of legal status. In the twentieth century, allopathic medicine was able to legally restrict the practice of medicine to doctors trained in medical school, because it argued that other practices were unscientific and hence dangerous. In 1910 the famous Flexner report criticized the state of medical education, and declared that all nonscientific schools should be closed. From that date onward, allopathic medicine reigned supreme. Midwives, homeopaths, herbalists, lay healers, chiropractors and anyone else who attempted to treat illness in its broadest sense could be prosecuted for practicing medicine without a license.

In 1977 Dana Ullman, a homeopath in Oakland, California was indicted for practicing medicine without proper credentials. His defense held that in practicing homeopathy he was doing something entirely different from conventional medicine, and was therefore not breaking any law. Because homeopathy had developed in a logical way, on the basis of different assumptions and observations, Dana Ullman had a powerful defense. Eventually his point of view prevailed and the state dropped its charges.

Jerry Green, a spokesman for holistic and nonallopathic practices, and Ullman's attorney, commented:

> Harris Coulter's books essentially show us that there is a scientific tradition that is focused on pathology, and there is one that hasn't. It has focused essentially on vital energy or life force. Homeopathy is the most recent expression of an empiric science . . .
>
> Bill Grey, who was going to be a witness in Dana's case, also was a respected Stanford graduate physician, who told me before I took Dana's case that he thought differently when he thought like a homeopath than when he thought like a physician.

Therefore, other forms of science can have validity—at least in some eyes. In our age of criticism concerning traditional Western medicine, this view is exceedingly appealing. It implies that not only are there social, political and cultural shortcomings in allopathic medicine, but other *scientific* alternatives as well. While conventional scientists maintain that this is a false notion, some consumers, legal authorities and philosophers are encouraging a pluralistic and changing perspective that encompasses more than the view taught in our medical schools. As we shall see, this is having a profound effect on the legal regulation of the new medicine.

chapter 3

Faith and the New Healers

Until the nineteenth century there was little distinction between faith and science in healing. Both clergy and healer acted as a conduit for the Will of God. If you were sick, you were ill in the spirit and mind as well as the body.

In the 1900's this belief changed. Healing was thrust out of the Church and into the laboratory. However, some faith healing did persist. At the end of the nineteenth century Lourdes became famous as a place of pilgrimage for the sick. This small town in southwestern France was catapulted into international fame because of the visions of 14-year-old Bernadette Soubirous, who felt that she saw the Virgin Mary at least 18 times between February 11 and July 16, 1858.

At first the Church and local officials doubted the peasant girl, and seemed embarrassed by the imposition of the supranormal into matters of healing. They placed Bernadette's visions, as well as the healing powers of Lourdes, under the most careful scrutiny. Eventually the piety and simplicity of Bernadette triumphed and Lourdes soon became known as a place where magical cures could be found. The spring that Bernadette discovered in the grotto of Massabielle was felt to run with waters that contained curative powers. A shrine was erected with crutches and other votive offerings on the walls, and millions flocked annually to be cured.

Although the sick flocked to Lourdes annually, the Church set several exceedingly stringent criteria for a cure: the illness had to be serious and difficult to treat, all medical therapy must have failed and the spiritual transformation must be total. There could be no relapse.

So strict were these criteria that of the millions of pilgrims who visited Lourdes, only 50 or 60 cures were accepted by the Church as truly miraculous. In an era of scientific discovery the Church did not want to be seen in competition with medicine—either in the eyes of physicians or the general public. Science had effectively thrust faith, at least religious faith, out of the healing setting.

One rejection of a cure at Lourdes was described by Brian Inglis in *The Case for Unorthodox Medicine:*

> [Jack] Traynor had been wounded by machine gun bullets during the Gallipoli landings. The nerves of his right arm had been severed, leaving it paralyzed, and he had become an epileptic from a head wound. In all he had been operated on by ten surgeons—including Sir Frederick Treves, who had been one of Edward VII's doctors. . . . At

> Lourdes, Traynor's paralysis and epilepsy left him; and in the follow-up by the same doctors three years later, as well as by members of the Lourdes bureau, all signs of atrophy had gone. He had no more fits; the hole in his skull had disappeared; and the doctors pronounced the cure "absolutely beyond and above the powers of nature"—an impression which must have been confirmed when Traynor decided to become a coal heaver. Yet in the eyes of the Church, Traynor's cure did not constitute a miracle. . . . (Inglis, 1965)

Traynor's story and the scrutiny with which healing is analyzed at Lourdes provide a dramatic example of the modern rejection of faith in healing. The Church clearly decided to leave healing to allopathy; in turn, modern medicine left spiritual matters to the clergy. The body and the spirit were seen as separate entities with separate ministries. Later, in this century, the American Medical Association began a program of more directed attacks on faith healers, quacks and unsubstantiated cures.

After more than 50 years the power of faith in healing was rediscovered by the medical community in the form of the *placebo effect.* The alternative healers became especially interested in this physiological and psychological process, calling it the "doctor within us." Norman Cousins, for instance, attributed this notion to Dr. Albert Schweitzer:

> The witch doctor succeeds for the same reason that the rest of us succeed. Each patient carries his own doctor inside him. They come to us knowing the truth. We are at our best when we give the doctor who resides within each patient a chance to work. (Cousins, 1979)

The new techniques of biofeedback, yoga and relaxation, which emphasized an individual's ability to control his or her own bodily functions, were readily adaptable to the placebo concept. Additional research pointed to the ability of placebos to produce pain relief through chemicals in the central nervous system called endorphins. These substances are known to be stimulated by conventional pain medications, acupuncture and "the doctor within us."

Many doctors still do not embrace this concept. They point to the fact that the placebo effect is difficult to test in a controlled, laboratory experiment. Moreover, different people react differently to the healing environment, and what enhances the faith of one person may not affect another. It is also extremely difficult, if not impossible, to devise placebo experiments on animals—the basis for biomedical research.

But alternative healers do not always feel bound by the rules of scientific investigation to prove that the placebo effect really works. Dr. Dorothy Waddell, head of the Alternative Therapies Unit at San Francisco General Hospital, puts it this way: "Our belief is that faith will shorten the treatment, and aid in the physiological reaction. . . . We [may] see dramatic improvements . . . but we understand that it doesn't constitute proof. . . ." Not all of the new healers, however, are as questioning as Dr. Waddell.

The new healers effectively mobilize the placebo response. They do this, first, by assuming that all of us have the potential for wellness within us. This is true even for patients with extremely serious illnesses, such as cancer. For instance, O. Carl Simonton, a radiation Oncologist, treats cancer patients by actively employing the body's own healing energies. By using his method of *imaging,* patients learn to conceptualize that the white blood cells of their body are attacking the cancer cells.

Simonton's work has been taken up by the alternative healing proponents because it actively involves the patient in cancer care. And while little proof for Simonton's method exists, it makes the statement that each of us has the power within us to be well, even in the face of serious illness. It actively enlists the faith of the healer and client in the notion that the body has an innate mechanism for wellness.

The alternative healers also try to draw on the lifestyle and cultural beliefs of their clients in the healing process. In many situations clients whose values differ from conventional American values encounter hostility from allopathic physicians. Their unorthodox nutritional practices, religious beliefs, extended family relationships, drug use and other behaviors often offend the physician, nurse and clinical staff. In contrast, the alternative healers have sought clients from among these subgroups of American society. Many of the healers are themselves unconventional—at least by comparison with the physicians of the allopathic system. In the alternative healing situation, both the unconventional client and practitioner begin at an advantage in mobilizing the placebo effect, because they accept and encourage each other's belief in alternate healing methods.

One-third of the clients at the Alternative Therapies Unit already either buy health foods, have had a prior interest in holistic health practices, or live alternative lifestyles. Other new medicine centers also draw heavily on people who are already disposed to unconventional methods. And since many of the new healers are themselves unconventional, they are able to be supportive of the values held by their clients.

However, it would be incorrect to think that all patients who seek alternative healing methods are unconventional in their lifestyle and beliefs. Often people come because all the traditional allopathic remedies have failed them. Sometimes they have found the side effects of allopathic medications unacceptable, or the available treatments promise only palliation of symptoms, without a cure.

Confidence in an alternative healer is built up in clients who either perceive a positive change in their health, or find the relationship with their healer rewarding. Not all people expect immediate results. But they are likely to be patient and accepting, even if the treatment is not immediately beneficial, provided there is warmth and understanding in their relationship with the healer. Even if the client is initially skeptical, the client's belief system can be activated when a healer sets up the right kind of communication.

Another way in which healers mobilize the placebo effect is by returning power to the patient. Kathleen Campbell, administrator of the Alternative Therapies Unit, puts it this way: "Our most successful patients are different in that they want to be in control. Sometimes they are exactly the kind of people who drive doctors crazy. They ask a lot of questions, such as 'What's in this medication that you are giving me?' or 'Why do I have to do this?' They are uppity patients, and uppity patients do really well here."

In therapies that involve behavior modification, such as biofeedback and relaxation, returning power to the patient is fundamental if the treatment is to work. People with stress-related illnesses—headaches, hypertension and chronic pain—need self-control in order to restore their belief in themselves and in their body. As Boston psychologist Dr.

Issac Greenberg says: "Biofeedback is more than just a behavior change. Real psychological changes occur too."

The Faith of the Client

The placebo effect begins with the client's belief that a treatment will work. In all probability every individual can respond to some extent to this belief, provided the conditions are established that promote the belief.

For instance, one group of surgeons attempted to investigate the power of warmth, professional counseling and understanding in the healing process of patients undergoing elective surgery. The experimental group was given pre- and postoperative attention by an anesthesiologist, who told the participants what to expect from the operation and the recovery period, as well as teaching them deep breathing techniques for relaxation. The control group went through the usual hospital routine.

The group that received the added attention, as well as positive reinforcement after the operation, left the hospital three days earlier and used only half the narcotic medication of the control group. Their healing was faster, and they had fewer complications. And because they left the hospital earlier, the cost of the procedure was reduced.

The positive effect of encouragement and the expectation of a beneficial result have also been investigated in the alternative healing setting. In a study done by researchers in the Department of Psychology at Queen's University in Kingston, Ontario, it was found that the expectation of a positive result could enhance the effect of acupuncture in relieving pain. This experiment tested whether it was important for the subjects to have a high expectation of a positive result or a moderate expectation in order for a positive result to occur, and whether such an expectation could be altered by the use of "bogus" acupuncture applied to the wrong points on the body.

The results showed that the expectation of a beneficial result, in the form of counseling prior to the experiment, greatly enhanced the outcome of the treatment. The subjects who received acupuncture in the wrong arm, but who were given a highly positive expectation that the treatment would work, had some small amount of pain reduction. Overall, however, the group that received both the positive encouragement and the appropriate treatment showed the greatest benefit. (Knox, 1979)

To take this kind of thinking one step farther, experimenters at the Behavioral Sciences Laboratory in Kansas City, Missouri examined the effect of "bogus" biofeedback signals (biofeedback signals that came from a tape that was completely independent of the actual responses of the subjects) on drug addicts who were withdrawing from methadone. One group of subjects received the correct biofeedback signal, while the other group received a tape of random responses. As it turned out, almost all of the subjects felt that they were receiving the correct biofeedback signals and reported benefits from the sessions.

As Dr. Isaac Greenberg points out, biofeedback produces a positive result in part because it enhances a person's own feeling of power in the healing process. The clients in the drug withdrawal study said that they had an increased sense of relaxation and an "out-of-body-sensation" that went along with a loss of space and time perception. They got a "high" which lasted for hours and helped with their withdrawal symptoms. In this case the expectation of a positive result was conveyed by participation in an alternative healing process—which by itself elicits faith in the healing method.

Dr. Dorothy Waddell described this kind of interaction in some of the patients treated with acupuncture at the Alternative Therapies Unit: "There is certainly a role that is played when the needle is inserted in terms of relief of pain or relaxation. That induces a mental change, as well as changes in different levels of the nervous system.

"The rest of the belief in the holistic system is based on experience. The reason that people get fired up is that they treat themselves, or they experience change. If they experience change that is vastly beyond what they got when they saw a doctor, then their belief gets attached to what they were doing. There is no doubt that these experiences happen, and are fairly profound."

Dr. Waddell's point, although hard to prove with conventional experiments, seems intuitively obvious. We don't necessarily have to begin with complete faith in either the healer or the healer's system, but over a period of time that belief must become cultivated.

Consequently, if there is a predisposition to accept the new healer and his methods, plus a movement toward better health, the placebo effect can become activated. Getting well is a *partnership in a process*—not something that the doctor does for the client, but something that the healer does *with* the client.

The Healer's Faith

The healer's faith is as important as the client's faith. The healer must believe in the method and have a commitment to its delivery to the patient. The alternative healers have had to struggle against the opposition of allopathic medicine and this has helped to activate their faith. Both chiropractors and osteopaths founded their professions in an environment of intense opposition from the established medical circles. Homeopathy was drummed out of the American medical scene at the turn of the century because it was deemed unscientific. Naturopathy remains on the fringes.

It is therefore in an environment of doubt and opposition that the alternative healers must practice their medicine. They maintain their faith through a profound conviction. Often they, like their clients, share a feeling of variance from the conventional values of American society. They also see severe limitations to the current allopathic system.

Professionals practicing alternative healing often claim to have experienced a profound cure that brought about their commitment. Dr. Edward Taub, for example, is a physician who left a traditional practice to go into holistic medicine. After completing a residency in pediatrics at the University of California at Irvine, he realized that many of his patients were not getting better. In his practice, 20% of his patients used about 50% of the total patient visits.

"[T]hese people, in so many ways, were lacking love," he says. "I began to readdress the definition of i-l-l as meaning I lack love."

Dr. Taub then went through a crisis in his own health. "I had developed a scotoma in my right eye. A scotoma is a black spot in the field of vision. This black spot took out about a quarter's worth of my vision.

"Traditional medicine does not know how this comes about, but is able to effectively cure it with laser beam surgery. I had been to several ophthalmologists, and they had referred me to several superspecialists at Stanford who wished to run a laser beam against the affected area of my retina. . . . I [decided] that I would not have the laser beam shot against my retina. I determined that in some way I would rid myself of this problem myself, and yet I hadn't the slightest idea about how to do it.

"A year ago at the Mandala Conference," continues Dr. Taub, "while walking through the corridor, I came across a lady who was emanating an exuberance and excitement that seemed to draw me toward her. I went up and introduced myself and she introduced herself to me as Olga Worrell [a new healer], while referring to me as 'Sonny.' She gazed at my eyes and said, 'Well, what is the matter with your eyes, Sonny, you have a black spot in there.' Now, a scotoma is a subjective thing to have in the sense that no one could see it or know it to be present, and this was mildly shocking, to say the least. My shock then grew to embarrassment as she said, 'Take off your glasses, Sonny.' And here we were with crowds walking by and I became intensely embarrassed and then she just put her hand over my eye and said something about, 'God is with you,' and I started feeling energy coming into my eye to such an extent that I felt elevated and experienced a sense of reverie. I talked to Barbara [Dr. Taub's wife and a registered nurse] about it and we both felt that I had had a most meaningful experience and had indeed met up with a phenomenal person.

"To make a long story short," concludes Dr. Taub, "one day after my encounter with Olga Worrell, I woke up from a deep sleep . . . and my scotoma was gone!" (Taub, 1980)

It is a mistake to think that rational thought moves all scientists—in fact, more intuitive kinds of realizations often produce the most profound internal changes. And of course, those who believe most strongly in what they do are the most likely to be able to convey a positive expectation to their clients. In other words, the healing partnership works most effectively when both the healer and the client have a deep faith in the healing process.

Faith in the Healing Environment

The final element in a healing system is the environment and interaction of the healer and the client toward promoting healing. It is in this that the alternative healers have made, perhaps, their most significant contribution.

They begin by accepting that the healing relationship is far more important than the specific healing technique. Norman Cousins aptly described this in an article he published in the *Journal of the American Medical Association* (1980) in which he told the stories of two patients who had cancer. One of these patients' physicians seemed to disregard the power of the patient's belief system, while the other chose to enhance that faith.

The first patient, a friend of Cousins, had undergone a biopsy for a suspected malignant tumor. Cousins recounted:

> There was no word from the physician for four days. The patient then received a certified letter in which the physician reported the findings of a carcinoma. There can be no doubt that, in sending a certified letter, the physician was able to create a legal record that would protect him against claims that the patient had not been fully informed. But neither can there be any doubt that the diagnosis of cancer, when delivered in the form of a certified letter, can have a catastrophic effect on the patient; it was akin to receiving an official eviction from life.

In contrast, Cousins then related another story that was reported to him by a patient who also was told he had a malignancy. Instead of a cold and defensive approach, this patient's physician attempted to employ the healing powers of the patient. The physician may not necessarily have seen himself as practicing alternative or holistic medicine, but the style was one of healer and client working together as co-equals, seeking health through medicine but using, as a foundation, the healing powers of the placebo effect.

> The physician called in the patient, who had cancer of the prostate, and spoke to him along the following lines (as reported to me by the patient).
>
> "I've got something serious to talk to you about. We've done a complete x-ray scan and it shows that your prostate cancer has spread. So we've both got a job to do. First let me tell you about my job, then I'll tell you about your job. If we both do our jobs well, you've got a good chance, a very good chance. My job is to try to knock out the male hormone. I'm going to give you estrogen. We may have surgery; as to that I'll be able to tell later.
>
> "Now let me tell you about your job. Whether I succeed depends to a large extent on how well you do your job. Your first job is to believe me when I say that the words cancer and death are not synonymous. Thousands of people overcome their cancers; thousands more stabilize their condition and live very effectively for many years. Then there are complete remissions that we in the medical profession cannot account for. We want to do everything possible to make you one of those remissions. One of your main enemies is terror. All that terror will do is to push you in the wrong direction. Conversely, your confidence in me and in yourself increases your chances. I want you to do everything you've always wanted to do. Have a good time. I want you to exercise

a robust will to live. Just know that we are partners and we'll give it our best shot." (Cousins, 1980)

The alternative healers have made the interaction of healer and client a foundation in their therapeutic practice. Rather than shrinking away from intimacy as the typical Western physician does, the new healers see this as an affirmation of the healer's role. However, some alternative healers do more than merely instill friendship into the healing environment. They attempt to communicate vital healing energy.

Dolores Krieger is a registered nurse who teaches at New York University. She is a proponent of therapeutic touch and the laying on of hands. As a part of the alternative healing movement, therapeutic touch emphasizes the conveyance of healing energy from the healer to the client. Ms. Krieger thinks that most anyone can transfer healing energy, but that it is a learned process—something that we must cultivate in ourselves to give to others. She believes that therapeutic touch is real in that it produces physiological changes that can be measured in terms of changes in the blood cell count and other physical parameters.

> I call this type of personalized interaction *therapeutic touch* simply because the term appears to be more acceptable to curriculum committees and other institutional bulwarks of today's society. However, in its long and ancient history it has been more descriptively called *laying-on of hands.* It is a mode of therapeutic intervention that seems to have been extant, according to histories of many literate cultures, throughout the world; however, because of its subjective nature it has been given little credence in modern technological society, whose scientific methodologies have been so deeply based on empirical evidence.
>
> I soon realized, however, that the touch in which I was

> interested was not simple physiological touch, but rather a humanized touch which conveyed an intent to help or to heal, and which was indeed suffused with this motivation. Moreover, the touch was that of a fairly healthy person whose ego structure was oriented towards serving the patient's needs, rather than his own needs. (Krieger, 1976)

The therapeutic environment that is set up by the alternative healers combines humanism, empathy and a return to a less technological approach to patient care. At San Francisco's Alternative Therapies Unit, for instance, the physical environment does not look like the typical hospital or physician's office. It is designed to make people feel comfortable, as if they were visiting someone's home. The Unit is situated in the oldest and least technical looking part of the hospital. The main room in which classes are held includes a fireplace, a carpet on the floor, windows that open, and a kitchen area with coffee and tea. The examination rooms have old fashioned floor-to-ceiling cupboards, and the staff often dresses in informal street clothes. There is little evidence of harried men and women in white coats with stethoscopes hanging from their necks, and laboratory equipment in the examination areas. The overall effect is one of de-emphasizing the technology of healing in favor of human needs. If the environment of the healing setting can convey a message, the one at the Alternative Therapies Unit is one that says, "You are the major force in getting better."

The Placebo in Unconventional Medicine

Until the last few years, the placebo effect, or faith, was looked upon with scorn by Western physicians. Doctors viewed people who responded to faith in the healing process as gullible, suggestible or naive. However, recent studies of people who respond to placebos have disproven this concept. There is no basic personality difference between those who respond to placebos and those who are unaffected. Moreover, pharmacological studies demonstrate that placebos catalyze the production of chemicals within the body in ways similar to those of drugs that are used to treat pain. In other words, placebos are real in their effect on the body as well as the mind.

Two obvious questions arise from this. First, why do the new healers employ the placebo response more effectively than the allopathic physician? Second, is there any value to the techniques of the new healers other than just the activation of the placebo effect?

The answer to both questions is unclear. The alternative healers and their techniques have not been subjected to careful scientific scrutiny. Their methods are often too new, and the healing environment is one that is notoriously hard to evaluate without bias, since in science as well as other areas, prejudices abound and tests are often designed to validate one's own preferences.

However, the alternative healers do seem to be more effective than allopathic physicians in enhancing the faith of their clients. People who are frustrated with the doctor-patient relationship that they have been accustomed to, or who have found that the kind of treatment they have been receiving is not acceptable are often motivated by alternative healing. And once these people see some movement or change for the better in themselves, they are further stimulated to believe in the particular alternative therapy they have been using.

There is a difference of style and approach between the new healer and the traditional physician, and this can be used to promote healing. For some people, however, allopathy also catalyzes the placebo effect. Our faith in our healers has been taught in our schools, through decades of Marcus Welby, Dr. Kildare and the public relations of an enormously powerful and wealthy medical establishment. So, even though modern doctors may eschew a belief in the placebo effect, they use it merely by their existence in a society that has been trained to think that the doctor is a healer. If we accept that in most situations about 30% to 35% of patients will respond to a nonspecific treatment by getting better, we can see that all healers are able to use the patient's inner healing mechanisms to advantage. However, it is advantageous to see the effect of the alternative healers in this area as promoting a new concept in medicine and forcing the allopathic system to make significant changes in its approach to both people and science.

The second question is whether the alternative healers do more than activate the placebo response, and this is even more difficult to answer. By and large, the new techniques are too new to evaluate completely. Moreover, the placebo effect is a confusing phenomenon, especially for the alternative therapies, which are often more subtle and probably more subject to social, motivational and emotional factors than is allopathic medicine. Techniques such as biofeedback and relaxation, for example, demand motivation on the part of the client that is more stringent than that required by most allopathic treatments. For this reason it is not realistic to decide on the efficacy of these treatments outside the social and personal context.

Furthermore, the healing powers of all practitioners are always greater in real life than in controlled studies. Statisticians call this "regression to the mean." In medicine this means that patients see their health providers when they are sickest—or, from a statistical point of view, at one end of the normal curve. The natural probability is that some short time later they will move back to the middle of the curve, back toward health.

Thus, the alternative methods, which do not fit easily into laboratory studies with cells, animals and chemical reactions, are even more difficult to look at critically; for while the physiologist can examine the effect of a drug on the heart by taking the organ out of an experimental animal's body, it is clearly not possible to do this with nutrition, exercise, meditation or even acupuncture.

However, there is some evidence for the usefulness of the new techniques. This will be the subject of the next chapters. We will identify those treatments that have potential independent of the placebo response, so that each of us, as consumers, can make better decisions about where to put our faith.

For now, we should keep in mind the words of William Osler, one of the founders of modern Western medicine:

> Far more important than what the physician does is the physician's belief and the patient's belief in what the physician does.

chapter 4

Evaluating the New Medicine: The Nondrug Therapies

Testing a medical theory or form of treatment is not easy. There is often an enormous variability in individual human response to both illness and treatment. The placebo effect may be elicited in one person but not in another. Sometimes a disease progresses virulently in one person but lies dormant or advances slowly in another. Spontaneous remission, which may occur independently of treatment, can further confuse matters.

Unfortunately, without large-scale testing, the alternative healing industry has often relied on anecdotal evidence —a healer claiming to have cured a particular illness; or a satisfied patient testifying to a miraculous recovery.

Anecdotes are often illustrative, but they are not proof.

Developing a science of investigation has been a slow process. In the West, rudimentary medical science began before the birth of Christ in Egypt and Greece. But medical tools were extremely limited. In the first century A.D. Galen founded the science of anatomy by making a study of the circulatory system. But Christianity intervened, and for the next 12 centuries dissection was prohibited. Medical science stood at a standstill.

From the fifteenth century onward, the Church's grip on science and learning began to loosen, and the study of dissection revived. Vesalius studied both animal and human cadavers, and advanced the work of Galen. Throughout the Renaissance, artists like DaVinci investigated the human form and made careful pictorial representations of the body. For the first time since the pre-Christian era the body was represented in nude form, indicating a willingness to study its shape, movement and function.

The science of investigation still proceeded extremely slowly—at least by modern standards. It was not until the end of the eighteenth century that physicians began to experiment with drugs and treatments in an organized fashion. In 1767 John Hunter gave himself both gonorrhea and syphilis by auto-injecting an infected penile discharge. Johannes Purkinje took an overdose of digitalis to study its side effects. Edward Jenner inoculated himself against smallpox. Samuel Hahnemann experimented with plant and animal substances and founded homeopathy. While primitive by modern standards, these early experiments showed a new desire to study medicine and to advance science. They represented the philosophy of a time of enlightenment applied to the human body.

Studying the effects of a particular treatment on a number of people was the next step in the experimental process. Unfortunately, many of the early clinical tests showed how research bias can create false hopes and promote useless therapies. For instance, in 1794 Dr. Benjamin Rush, probably the most famous American physician of the Colonial period (and for whom the Rush Medical College in Chicago is named), published a study of bloodletting as a treatment for yellow fever. In one day he bled 100 patients, and afterwards triumphantly declared his success by noting that not a single patient had died. Dr. Rodney Nelson of the Abraham Lincoln School of Medicine at the University of Illinois analyzes the pitfalls of Dr. Rush's approach:

> His description of the effectiveness of bloodletting for yellow fever remains a classic example of the triumph of optimism and passion over reason and scientific principles . . . he reports no controls except for the implication that some yellow fever patients not treated by him died. There is no record of attempting to standardize conditions, and follow-up could not have exceeded twenty-four hours. In short, it seems that in his anxiety to be of help, Rush persuaded himself that his treatments were safe and effective. (Nelson, 1979)

In the post-World War II era, clinical tests have undergone major refinements in an attempt to eliminate this bias. Today scientists agree that large-scale, organized clinical testing of a treatment is essential. We need only to look at the history of such medical disasters as Thalidomide[T] and DES (drugs which produced birth defects) to see that insufficient testing presents enormous potential risks.

Clinical tests are first performed on animals. These

studies look for both therapeutic benefit and harmful side effects. If the animal studies show promise, small-scale testing is performed on humans.

If these studies demonstrate promise, then more tests that compare the new treatment to a treatment of known effectiveness are done. Finally, additionally refined studies are set up to examine the effectiveness of the treatment on the many patients that may be affected by a particular disease. For instance, a cancer treatment may be effective only if the disease is discovered at a particular stage. It might be useless and unethical to apply this treatment to patients who do not fit into this category.

Furthermore, studies must check for bias on the part of the researcher and the patient. These "blind" conditions (single-blind if only the patient is unaware of the type of treatment; double-blind if both doctor and patient are unaware) control for the placebo effect of expectation. In the double-blind study the healer must be equally enthusiastic about all the types of treatment being tested. This is usually the best way to eliminate prejudice on the part of the healer.

Alternative healers frequently report studies in which the healer is permitted to be the advocate of a given form of treatment. When this is permitted there is an enormous potential for introducing bias and catalyzing the placebo effect.

An example of this can be seen in one study concerning migraine headache, relaxation and biofeedback. Patients who were placed on a waiting list and told that they would be treated at a later date noted a *40% reduction* in the frequency of headache attacks. The role of expectation, although certainly a nonspecific factor in medical therapy, is a potentially potent variable. Double-blind studies are designed to eliminate, or at least minimize, this type of effect.

The Ethics of Research

In the eighteenth and nineteenth centuries medical scientists usually tested their theories on themselves and their coworkers. Perhaps this was due to a general skepticism on the part of the public. Science was not a household word, and most people were still illiterate. To some degree this probably represented a medical *machismo*. Risky as it was, it helped protect the public from new and untried treatments that could be dangerous.

After World War II and the Nuremberg trials, a code of ethics for medical experimentation was created. Ethical research, the Nuremberg code said, must be intended to obtain useful medical information, and a planned study is necessary to obtain such information. Wherever possible, research should be conducted on animals, and always designed to minimize human suffering. Point number six perhaps summarizes the intent of the Nuremberg code: "The degree of risk should never exceed the value to humanity."

Little in the code provides an argument against the experimental validation of alternative therapies. For the most part, however, the alternative therapies are inherently safe. The nondrug therapies such as biofeedback, meditation, relaxation training, Rolfing and Feldenkrais (body-awareness therapies) do not invade the body with drugs or surgery. Even homeopathy, which administers vegetable and mineral substances as remedies, does so in extremely dilute form. Acupuncture, although involving the insertion of fine needles, is rarely associated with dangerous side effects.

Two sticky points do arise with regard to the Nuremberg code. First, it may not often be easy to plan initial experiments with an alternative therapy on laboratory animals. Certainly this applies to biofeedback, meditation and progressive relaxation training. Second, there may be a problem in trying unproven treatments in serious illnesses for which a known allopathic treatment is effective. For instance, it is questionable whether anyone should stop taking blood pressure medication prior to entering a study comparing medication to biofeedback in hypertension. This concern would also apply to vitamin or dietary treatments of cancer such as laetrile. For although many forms of chemotherapy are both extremely toxic and of uncertain effectiveness, a completely untried therapy poses a grave risk. Perhaps, if people are sufficiently aware of the alternatives, fully informed consent can satisfy the ethical questions.

In any case there is an immediate need to study the effectiveness of the new alternative therapies. There is nothing ethical or humanitarian about touting unproven methods of treatment in advertisements and the popular press. Similarly, practitioners who claim the effectiveness of a type of treatment without subjecting it to scientific testing, or submitting their claims to professional analysis are guilty of hucksterism. Dr. Jerome Schofferman of the Alternative Therapies Unit of San Francisco General Hospital says: "What bothers me is that I have asked a number of people [alternative healers] to show me in their records any . . . case of someone proven to have cancer, and who has been cured by their treatment. I have not seen one case, and I know that I can produce more than that from spontaneous remissions, whatever that means. I know that the people who are reputable do not claim to have magic and have looked at their results and will share them with you."

Clearly the alternative healing industry would be serving its own best interest to endorse good clinical trials.

Testing Alternative Therapies

Clinical investigation takes money, often large sums of it. In 1945 the National Institutes of Health had a budget of $701,800 to fund research. By 1965 this figure had mushroomed to $436,600,000. In the 1970's the money rose into the billions, with additional funds available through private foundations and drug companies.

By contrast, almost no money has been provided for the study of alternative therapies. For instance, in 1973 and 1974 the Department of Health, Education and Welfare awarded a paltry $2 million for research into chiropractic. Yet during this time chiropractors saw more than *100 million* patient visits. One would think that the government would be more interested in validating or refuting treatment that appeared to enjoy such widespread public support.

A difficulty that arises in testing alternative therapies in good clinical trials is isolating single methods of treatment. Often alternative therapy patients try a number of types of treatment for a single problem. They may simultaneously alter their diet, exercise, meditate and receive acupuncture. While this approach may make sense for the patient, it can cloud the evidence obtained in a clinical trial, where only one hypothesis should be tested at a time.

Nevertheless some standard needs to be developed. Consumers have a right to know what to expect from a particular type of therapy. This includes information about the effectiveness of a treatment, the type of person most likely to benefit from it, and the possible side effects of the treatment. Individual case histories, anecdotal stories and claims by proponents never answer these questions. It takes testing on a large scale in well-thought-out studies.

Biofeedback

Of all the new therapies, biofeedback has probably been the most tested. In part this is a result of its historical development. The original research into biofeedback came out of the laboratory. On the basis of earlier work by behavioral psychologists and physiologists, it was natural and easy to test the biofeedback system. One could hook up clients to a feedback sensor and record their responses. The information from such a signal-and-response system could be interpreted scientifically.

Biofeedback is also, in some respects, the ultimate modern placebo therapy. Early in its development it enjoyed an enormous amount of publicity in the popular media. This coverage biased both clients and practitioners to expect positive results. Otherwise skeptical doctors, who might have been reluctant to suggest meditation or progressive relaxation, referred patients for biofeedback therapy.

Moreover, the biofeedback machines themselves enhanced the placebo response by adding glamor to the therapy. The light and sound signals of these instruments symbolized the application of engineering technology to medicine. In a machine age, the technology of biofeedback caught the imagination of enthusiasts already used to remarkable advances in such other areas of science as computers, space flight and telecommunications.

Not surprisingly, the initial reports of the usefulness of

biofeedback were confused with the optimism of overzealous proponents, and biofeedback enjoyed a rather uncritical beginning. It was hoped that it would be a fast form of treatment. Many hoped that in a few sessions a variety of medical problems from headache to anxiety would respond to the treatment. People were looking for easy answers to complex medical problems.

The "alpha state" that received popular publicity is an example of this expectation. The alpha rhythm is an 8- to 12-cycle-per-second brain wave that is recorded on the electroencephalograph (EEG). The alpha state was thought to represent the relaxed but intensely aware mental and emotional state that yogis and Zen masters attain through meditation.

Alpha training was applied to a number of medical disorders, including vascular and migraine headache, chronic pain, psychiatric disturbances and drug withdrawal. However, alpha training, when used in a controlled study, did not prove to be effective. It also did not produce the heightened state of awareness and inner peace of the Buddhist monk or Zen master. There was, in reality, no quick way to attain enlightenment through alpha training.

As research continued, it became questionable whether an alpha state actually existed. The brain is not a uniform organ in its functioning; parts of the cortex could be in alpha while other parts might be in other rhythms, since the EEG registers a *summation* of billions of firing neurological cells. Moreover, the autonomic nervous system that controls such basic body functions as the heart rate, breathing rate, temperature and digestion is deeper within the brain substance than the cortex. The centers that control these functions are not directly registered by the EEG machine; instead, their neurological activity is filtered through the cortex. The control that experienced meditators exert over their autonomic nervous system is therefore probably more complex than that which can be tested or trained using the alpha rhythm. In short, if there is an alpha state, current research has not been successful in demonstrating its use in medical therapy or in attaining heightened awareness. Furthermore, the state of calm that many people perceived during alpha training could also be obtained by sitting in a comfortable chair in a quiet room and relaxing. Similar results have been seen when people listen to restful music for 20 minutes. Bogus biofeedback (responses that are not related to the performance of the patient) can induce a sense of inner calm. (Blanchard, 1979; Cohen, 1977)

EEG biofeedback has shown some potential in treating epilepsy. This form of training is not a substitute for medication, but is an adjunct to standard medical therapy. It helps epileptics reduce the frequency of seizures, and may aid in reducing the overall medication needed. This application of biofeedback is an example of how very specific situations may be amenable to biofeedback training.

The electromyograph (EMG machine), which records muscle activity through electrodes placed on the skin, is another popular treatment. As with the EEG, EMG biofeedback has been tried in a variety of disorders including headache, anxiety, facial pain, cerebral palsy and paralysis.

The rationale behind EMG training in tension headache is based on the hypothesis that these headaches are created by tension in the muscles of the scalp, neck or face. Training often employs monitoring tension levels in the *frontalis* muscle of the forehead. Controlled studies, however, have not demonstrated that this treatment reliably reduces the frequency or severity of tension headaches.

EMG training has been most promising as part of a

total program of rehabilitation for people who have suffered injury to their nervous system. After a spinal cord injury or a stroke, for instance, the normal nervous system feedback about the position and function of parts of the body may be interrupted. The EMG helps persons with this problem to retrain those parts of the body that have been affected. Paralysis, facial spasms, torticollis (holding of the neck in an abnormal and rigid position), disordered movements, and fecal incontinence may respond to EMG training. However, the training process is slow and painstaking, and should only be employed in conjunction with physical therapy, occupational therapy, skilled nursing and medical care and psychological counseling.

Biofeedback and Hypertension

Hypertension, or high blood pressure, affects at least 15% of the adult population in the United States. It is an important risk factor in stroke, heart disease and many of the other serious illnesses that affect millions.

The biofeedback training of persons with hypertension, so that they may reduce their own blood pressure, is relatively easy to perform; however, the results have not been conclusive. This is another area in which initially optimistic claims have been modified by more detailed investigation.

Hypertension is, in reality, an extremely complex medical disease. Emotional tension, exercise, diet and attitude all play an enormous role in this disorder. For instance, a cup of coffee can raise the blood pressure by as much as 14%. Emotional stress may also elevate the blood pressure. On the other hand, exercise, when performed on a regular basis, can lower blood pressure.

Over 50 years ago David Ayman, a Boston physician, studied the effects of placebo in modifying the symptoms of hypertension. He gave hypertensive patients a few drops of dilute hydrochloric acid (a placebo), and found that 82% of the patients in the study reported a reduction in such symptoms as headache, nervousness, insomnia, palpitations and vomiting.

In 1956, Dr. William Goldring, a New York physician, performed an even more dramatic demonstration of this placebo effect. He used an electron gun that emitted a loud noise and a bluish spark. Each patient in the study was treated by a nurse who spent time getting to know the person, and who told them that the gun therapy had been proven to reduce blood pressure. During the treatment periods she pointed the gun at the patient and discharged the spark.

In a group of hospital patients, 6 out of 9 had blood pressure reductions that averaged 39 mmHg systolic and 28 mmHg diastolic. Similar results were obtained in outpatients. During the study the patients also noted subjective improvement in such symptoms as headache, fatigue, dizziness, chest pain and nervousness that they associated with their hypertension. While we do not know whether these people made changes in their diet, exercise habits or emotional problems during the spark-gun study, the results point to the complex nature of hypertension and the potential role of belief in its cure.

Thus, in analyzing the value of biofeedback training in treating hypertension, placebo factors have been shown to play a role. However, reducing a subject's blood pressure during a study does not mean that it will stay lowered after the study ends. Nor does it mean that during the study period, the blood pressure will stay down when the subject is out of the laboratory. And how does one know whether it is biofeedback that produced the blood pressure reduction?

The most promising use of biofeedback in treating hypertension has been in conjunction with relaxation training or meditation. Here the biofeedback response helps people train themselves to appreciate when their blood pressure is reduced, and they use this training to clue themselves into their physiological state and to correlate this state with their feelings.

There is little evidence to support using biofeedback as a single method of treatment. It may be a useful tool in conjunction with an overall plan that includes diet modification, exercise, relaxation and medication (where necessary). With successful training, biofeedback may help people reduce their need for medication. In some situations they may even eventually cease to require medication, but this is likely to be a slow process. In general it would be unwise to abruptly stop one's medication and substitute biofeedback.

Potentially serious medical problems, like hypertension, demand sensitive treatment by practitioners; and people who seek alternative therapies (like biofeedback) should not expect easy and miraculous results. Biofeedback training and the other alternative modalities demand that people be willing to make many changes in their lifestyle.

Meditation, Relaxation, and Autogenic Training

Like biofeedback, these methods involve learning to control one's own autonomic nervous system. Like biofeedback, they are not exclusive forms of therapy. They can be learned in conjunction with biofeedback or used while making changes in diet, exercise, or taking most prescription medications.

Meditation is the oldest of these methods. In the Orient, Buddhist monks, Japanese Zen masters and others have meditated for more than 2,500 years in order to attain spiritual enlightenment, a relaxed body state, and oneness with God. More recently, in the West, meditation gained popularity as a secular means of relaxing and heightening spiritual awareness. In the 1960's the Beatles and the media made Transcendental Meditation and the Maharishi Mahesh Yogi household words. Businessmen, housewives, students and counterculture enthusiasts began to meditate.

Medical scientists also became interested in meditation. When masters of the art were studied by physiologists, it was discovered that these meditators had reduced heart and breathing rates, a lowered blood pressure and a reduced oxygen consumption indicative of a lowered metabolic rate. Meditation was considered to be a type of "hypometabolic state" in which the mind and the body were in a condition of pleasurable repose.

Moreover, meditation is relatively easy to learn, is safe, and requires no medical technology. It can be performed in any quiet place. Some people even claim that they can meditate while riding the subway or during their lunch break at the office. If one sits in a quiet place, in a comfortable position, and repeats a simple phrase, one begins to get into the meditative state. In some disciplines the phrase that is repeated is called a "mantra." You can also begin to meditate by becoming aware of your rhythmic breathing. The exact method or mantra that is used is relatively unimportant. With continued practice, more profound and deeper meditative states can be attained. However, it is erroneous to think that everyone can attain the level of the

Zen master or Buddhist monk. This takes training and a lifetime of dedication.

Nevertheless, seeing the physiological effects of meditation, researchers immediately appreciated its potential application to a variety of medical problems including irritability, depression, insomnia, phobias, chronic pain and hypertension. In addition, since meditators report increased feelings of self-control, self-actualization and harmony with the environment, meditation seemed to be a method for achieving the high-level wellness sought by the holists.

Research into meditation has been limited in its application to medical disorders. Few studies have been performed which distinguish nonspecific effects (placebo) from those specific to meditation. Can one, for instance, get similar results by relaxing in a quiet place? Moreover, there have not been serious attempts to compare meditation to psychological counseling, a regular exercise program, or empathy and support from friends in the treatment of emotional disorders.

There are many anecdotal reports of individual improvement in emotional disorders after meditation. During the 1960's and 1970's many people tried meditation to relieve stress, anxiety and other neurotic problems. But these anecdotal reports do not check for the normal ebbing and flowing of neuroticism. Moreover, since people often try new techniques when they are at a personal low point, improvement may result from regression upon the mean—the effect of "tincture of time," in which one begins to feel better after the crisis has passed. This concept of regression on the mean applies in such illnesses as the flu and muscle strains as well as in many emotional disorders; the body has an internal mechanism for correcting itself.

As with biofeedback, time and testing modified the initial claims of the proponents of meditation. Meditation has, for instance, demonstrated some usefulness in the treatment of insomnia. It may not be better than relaxation training, but it can help reduce the time it takes to get to sleep. It should be employed in conjunction with psychological counseling, behavioral therapy and support.

Meditation has also been used in the treatment of hypertension. With experience, meditation does train one to lower one's blood pressure. This does not necessarily mean that the blood pressure remains low throughout the day, but it certainly can be reduced during the meditation period. As with biofeedback, such training is a useful adjunct to an overall program that employs medication, counseling, diet and exercise.

Meditation is extremely safe. Occasional reports have appeared in the medical literature of people who have experienced psychosomatic illnesses, depression, hallucination, schizophrenic breakdown and suicide after beginning to meditate. Whether this occurs coincidentally to the meditation or as a result of it is not known. If it is a result of meditation, it probably occurs when inexperienced people meditate for excessively long periods. These adverse psychological symptoms may then result from stimulus deprivation and isolation. For this reason, people who begin a meditation program for emotional disturbances should do so in conjunction with a trained therapist. In such a setting the meditation becomes one part of an overall effort at solving the emotional problem. When the millions of people throughout the world who meditate daily are considered, the incidence of potentially harmful reactions to meditation is extremely small.

Relaxation training, sometimes called progressive relaxation, is another method of controlling one's autonomic nervous system. In the 1920's and 1930's Dr. Edmund Jacobsen, a Chicago physician and physiologist, developed this tool from the concept that one's muscles cannot be relaxed if the mind is tense. He found that by learning to alternately relax and tense major muscle groups, people could induce an overall state of relaxation. This relaxed state is a variation on meditation. The subject's heart rate, breathing, blood pressure and emotional tension are reduced. The mind and body enter a state of internal repose.

One can progressively relax with various techniques. One set of exercises begins with the client lying in a quiet room, with eyes closed. The client starts by making a fist and saying silently, "I clench my fist, I hold the tension (for about 15 or 20 seconds) and then I relax my hand."

The exercise is then repeated for the muscles of the arms, shoulders, face, abdomen, back, buttocks, feet and legs. The more one practices, the more one is capable of rapidly and readily inducing a state of spontaneous and complete relaxation. After finishing the exercise routine, the client lies in a state of pleasurable repose and the autonomic nervous system functions at a lowered level.

Autogenic training is another form of programmed relaxation. In this method one lies on the floor and imagines the parts of the body becoming heavy and warm. For instance, you can begin by saying to yourself, "My right hand is heavy," followed by, "My left hand is heavy," and so on through the various parts of the body. After imagining the heaviness, you imagine warmth: "My right hand is warm," then "My left hand is warm" and so on. At the end of the exercise you imagine that "My heartbeat is calm and regular" and "My body breathes by itself." Again, the result is a toning down of the autonomic nervous system. Like meditation and progressive relaxation, autogenic training can be performed while riding the bus to work or during lunch break at the office. The training is only a tool, and as such is very much like the mantra of meditation or the muscle tensing and relaxing of progressive relaxation.

Like meditation, relaxation training has been applied to the treatment of hypertension. Since some authorities suggest that hypertension at least partly results from excess stimulation of the sympathetic nervous system (the adrenalin-secreting portion of the nervous system, which heightens alertness, muscle tension and other body functions in the "flight or fight" response), it was hoped that relaxation training would be an effective form of therapy. The low blood pressure of yogis and Zen masters seemed to support this concept.

At Stanford University, hospital patients were given a simple form of relaxation training. The patients lay on the floor, breathed deeply, imagined themselves in a pleasurable environment and relaxed their major muscle groups. They performed this training three times a day, and by the fifth day were noted to have significantly lowered blood pressure. However, it is known that resting in the hospital will reduce blood pressure in most people, so that it was important to extend this study to outpatients.

In Britain, Dr. Chandra Patel performed studies to compare relaxation training to yoga meditation and biofeedback. He found that all three of the methods could reduce blood pressure, but that the yoga group had the best results. When he trained the relaxation group to perform the yoga, he found that they could further reduce their blood pressure. And when he retested the subjects 6 months later, he found that their lowered blood pressure had remained low. (Patel, 1975, 1977)

Relaxation therapy has been studied in other medical disorders. In a study performed in Israel, relaxation training helped people reduce elevated levels of serum cholesterol by about 10%. Although the study was done on only a small number of people, the lowered cholesterol appeared to be related to a decrease in sympathetic nervous system activity, i.e., stress reduction. Thus, stress may increase the breakdown of fatty acids and triglycerides, and eventually liberate cholesterol into the bloodstream. (Cooper, 1979)

Relaxation training has also been tested in the treatment of insomnia. At Rutgers University, in New Jersey, researchers attempted such a test while seeking to control for the placebo effect. The placebo group of subjects received additional attention from the research team and were taught to expect positive results, but did not perform the relaxation exercises. The group that learned the relaxation exercises was able to reduce the time needed to fall asleep. However, these positive results were found only in the group most severely affected by insomnia (those who needed more than 90 minutes to fall asleep each night). The group with more moderate insomnia was more likely to respond to the placebo therapy. (Carr-Kaffashan, 1979)

As already noted, the therapies discussed above are not useful substitutes for existing allopathic treatments. They are, however, complicated by few possibly adverse side effects, and can be employed as additional treatments with any conventional treatment. All of these methods demand time and effort from the client. They are not "quick fixes." Like biofeedback, they must be practiced regularly. There is no fast and easy way to train one's autonomic nervous system to function like that of the Zen master.

The contribution of the placebo effect in meditation, relaxation training, and autogenic training is still unknown. A positive expectation of beneficial results on the part of both the therapist and the client seems to be an important factor in the success of the technique that is used. Certainly this will help motivate people to perform their meditation or relaxation on a regular basis. There is nothing wrong with the contribution of the placebo effect in this regard. Anything that helps promote a positive change is a valuable adjunct to alternative or allopathic treatment.

Chiropractic

More than any other alternative form of therapy, chiropractic has been shrouded by mystery and controversy. Since its early beginnings, chiropractors have claimed the ability to care for every human ailment. In the 1920's chiropractic established hospitals in the United States that took pride in treating the most difficult cases, ranging from infectious diseases to psychiatric disorders. Yet chiropractic never sought to prove its theories or demonstrate its effectiveness through the usual form of clinical investigation characteristic of modern science. The paucity of evidence published concerning the effectiveness of chiropractic has put a cloud over its attempts to gain credence and respectability in medical circles.

The theoretical basis of chiropractic further encases the sense of mystery and uncertainty of this practice. Chiropractors claim that small displacements of the vertebrae, called *subluxations,* entrap and damage the nerves of the body.

These may become responsible for almost any kind of illness, from back pain to disorders of the internal organs. Unfortunately, these "subluxations" can rarely be seen on an X ray by conventional physicians, and have never been shown to correlate with disease when cadavers are examined at autopsy. Thus, the "subluxation" that chiropractors refer to appears to be largely a theoretical construct accepted primarily by chiropractors. Usually, chiropractors treat patients who have normal X rays and a normal bone structure—at least by allopathic standards.

Despite this controversial underpinning, patients have flocked to chiropractors, apparently satisfied to accept, as an article of faith, the explanation that is offered. Moreover, there is no unusual gullibility or lack of education in these clients. Chiropractic patients are no different from allopathic patients in social class, in the frequency or recurrence of their problem, in the severity of how they perceive their illness or in their tendency toward self-treatment. For decades, and in many countries throughout the world, chiropractors have treated intelligent people, whose principal common characteristic seems to be pain, illness and an inability to obtain relief from traditional allopathic treatment.

The fact that chiropractors often treat a variety of medical problems unrelated to the back, skeleton or muscles has been a thorny concern to allopathy. In a Canadian inquiry into chiropractic, researchers found that 61% of chiropractors said that they regularly treated gynecological problems. Fifty-seven percent said that they treated headaches. Seventy-eight percent said that they routinely prescribed vitamin and dietary supplements, and an even greater number reported that they prescribed dietary regimens. Thirty-seven percent said that they treated psychological problems such as nervousness, anxiety, neurosis and depression. (Mills, 1966)

The functioning of chiropractors as generalists and family medical practitioners may reflect the flight of patients away from traditional medical care. In the United States the number of family physicians decreased after World War II, while the number of medical specialists greatly increased. Chiropractors apparently saw the need to become family-care givers and decided to fill it. This was not necessarily based on a rational consumer choice, but on the failure of conventional medicine to provide the empathetic, hands-on care associated with the family doctor.

In 1977 the Australian government published a committee report on chiropractic. They said that they had failed to find any scientific basis for chiropractic therapy, and had been unable to find a single truly scientific study that analyzed the effectiveness of chiropractic treatment. As one might expect, this report was received with considerable criticism in chiropractic circles. In January of 1978 a more extensive Commission on Inquiry into Chiropractic was formed.

Since then a number of clinical tests have been performed to test chiropractic efficacy. In one of these studies (Parker, 1978) chiropractic manipulation was compared to conventional mobilization of the neck (moving the head through its normal range of motion) and placebo in the treatment of migraine headache. After 6 months of study, each of the treatment groups reported improvement in their condition; chiropractic was found to be no more advantageous than either the neck exercises or the placebo. When the study was continued, to follow the patients over 20 months, those who initially reported improvement continued to be improved while those who did not initially respond did not experience a change in the frequency or severity of their migraine attacks. (Parker 1978, 1980)

In chiropractic, as in the other alternative therapies, there appears to be a link between the expectation of a positive result and actually obtaining benefit. Sixty-two percent of the subjects in the migraine headache study who were initially optimistic about the potential positive effect of treatment reported either a marked diminution of their attacks or in some cases a cure. On the other hand, only one-third of those who were initially pessimistic reported benefiting from the treatment. Since other studies report that chiropractors commonly explain to their patients that their treatment is going to be effective, this may point to the importance of the placebo effect in obtaining patient improvement.

Similar results have been seen in the few studies that have compared chiropractic to conventional therapy for back pain. This is an area in which allopathic medicine is notoriously unreliable and ineffective. Yet while chiropractors probably treat more low back pain than any other single problem, they have not proven that they can be of help. Manipulation has not been shown to be more effective than rest or treatment with a corset. Chiropractic manipulation may help people feel better more rapidly, but when patients are followed up in the weeks after treatment, similar results are obtained with other methods.

However, chiropractors probably benefit from the placebo effect in this area of treatment. They are known for treating back pain. They are better than allopaths in explaining to clients what is going on in their bodies and what to expect from the treatment, and they have the psychological benefit of producing the "click" or "snap" sound that patients often associate with an effective treatment. Moreover, chiropractors present themselves as being competent, understanding and enthusiastic about the likelihood of curing the client's problem. In one study they were reported to have said such things as: "You have come to the right place," and "I can help your problem best." Of course, these are essential elements of the healer-client relationship that catalyzes the placebo effect. (Buerger, 1975; Doran, 1975)

The history of their conflict with allopaths may also help chiropractors in the treatment of certain patients. As people have become increasingly suspicious and critical of traditional physicians, the status of chiropractors, who have fought the medical establishment, has increased.

For years allopathic medicine has tried to convince the public that seeing a chiropractor is potentially dangerous. They claim that as primary care medical providers, chiropractors have, at best, a limited form of medical training. Allopaths point out that chiropractic students do not have access to conventional teaching hospitals, where the bulk of an allopathic physician's training and experience is obtained. They argue that because of this limited training, there is a potential for the chiropractic physician to fail to recognize a serious but potentially treatable illness.

Chiropractic does not recognize this deficiency in its training. In 1978 the Council on Chiropractic Education issued a "Position/Policy Paper" which declared:

> The purpose of his [the doctor of chiropractic] education is to prepare the doctor of chiropractic as a primary health-care provider. As a portal-of-entry to the health-delivery system, the chiropractic physician must be well

> trained to diagnose, including, but not limited to, spinal analysis; to care for the human body in health and disease; and to consult with, or refer to, other health-care providers.

The last point has been a politically difficult one for the chiropractic profession. Organized medicine has been unwilling, until very recently, to accept professional referrals from chiropractors, and for a long time the allopathic establishment asked that physicians refrain from working with chiropractic patients. Despite this negative approach, little good evidence has been published that documents missed diagnoses or harm to the general public inflicted by chiropractors. As times have changed, and with the growth of chiropractic, organized medicine has rescinded its earlier admonitions that allopaths should not work along with chiropractic.

There have been reports in the medical literature of rare but documented injury resulting from chiropractic manipulation. These cases have involved paralysis and occasionally death resulting from excessive manipulation. The first report of such an injury appeared in the *Journal of the American Medical Association* in 1925. A severe dislocation of the neck in this case resulted in the death of the patient. The cause of death was perhaps secondary to interruption of the blood supply entering the brain. Interestingly, a similar report appeared in 1977 in the *Archives of Neurology,* resulting from injury during a yoga exercise.

The public has a right to know whether it is the infectious enthusiasm, positive skills of interpersonal communication, "hands-on" quality of chiropractic care or actual manipulation by the chiropractor that produces positive results. The public should also be assured that chiropractors have a legitimate claim to treat illnesses unrelated to the skeleton, like gynecological disorders, psychological problems, nutritional deficiencies and the myriad of other illnesses normally treated by allopathic methods.

Body Therapies

In recent years alternative therapies have focused interest on reorganization of the body through movement and postural therapies. Two methods, Feldenkrais and Rolfing, have become popular for retraining individuals with chronic structural problems of the skeleton. Interestingly, both methods developed independently from conventional physical therapy, which is a supportive discipline to orthopedic surgery and rehabilitative medicine.

Rolfing was conceived by Dr. Ida Rolf, an organic chemist at the Rockefeller Institute in New York, and whose method has been called *structural integration.* Feldenkrais was developed by an Israeli physicist, Dr. Moishe Feldenkrais. The Feldenkrais method has been described as *functional integration.* While neither discipline claims to make conventional allopathic diagnoses, both have often been applied to a variety of structural ailments of the skeleton and muscular system.

Rolfing focuses on realigning posture. It hypothesizes that stress and our upright posture are the basis for profound structural disorganization of the body. With advancing years, people typically slump, stoop and become imbalanced. The result of this is distortion of the fascia (the connective tissues of the body) and permanent postural injury. In some cases, accidents initiate this injury, which is then further aggravated by emotional factors. Thus, skeletal problems are seen as resulting from both psychological and physical imbalances. Society, in creating internal stress, creates *tightness* in the body and personality.

Rolfing stretches the body to release the chronic tightness of the fascia. While not necessarily dangerous, it may be associated with pain and soreness. For some people, this stretching has the psychological effect of producing release from emotional tension.

The Feldenkrais method differs from the Rolfing technique in that it involves *relearning* disorganized or misused patterns of movement. Feldenkrais does not create pain or soreness in the skeletal structures through stretching movement; the emphasis is on retraining one's movement to produce awareness of chronic patterns of misuse of the body. Often these patterns have been developed and reinforced since childhood, although they may occur in response to a traumatic physical and psychological injury.

In both Rolfing and Feldenkrais there is an interest in the emotional counterpart to physical deformity, and a political and sociological connection with the forces that create emotional and physical imbalance. This is an element lacking in traditional physical therapy, which focuses mainly on the physical factors relating to illness (stroke, cerebral palsy, traumatic injury, etc.). Rolfing posits that the contractions in the fascia are symptoms of a stressful society that promotes emotional "tightness." Feldenkrais links disability, in part, to the need to succeed in competitive Western society. Yochanan Rywerant, a pupil of Feldenkrais, writes:

> Most commonly, the way in which [persons with physical or psychological difficulties] will attempt to improve their level of performance is by trying harder, striving to do

> better, increasing one's effort, using "will power," or by repetitive exercises—all with the hope that the results will ultimately emerge during the actual performance, contest, or concert.
>
> It is important to be aware of the philosophical assumptions underlying this common attitude, assumptions that are inherent in our Western culture and our educational practices. We hear the tutor saying: "Imitate a model, try hard, be serious, train both your will power and endurance, practice over and again—otherwise you will fail." The underlying religious assumptions seem to say, "You are a sinner and will get your reward only the hard way: your ongoing punishment is for all of your life to be an unrelenting examination process, demanding your constant self-sacrifice."
>
> But despite the commonality of this view, the results of such a procedure are unusually disappointing: very few persons ever succeed in improving their general abilities merely through routine striving. (Rywerant, 1977)

These philosophical and political underpinnings are consistent with the basic tenets of the alternative therapies, which hold that the root of many disorders are social, political and emotional stress. Both Rolfing and Feldenkrais express concepts that are rarely voiced in allopathy, yet which have increasingly become recognized as basic to the origins of disease.

There is little scientific evidence to support either the theoretical formulations or clinical effectiveness of either Rolfing or Feldenkrais. Both Ida Rolf and Moishe Feldenkrais have excelled as teachers, spreading their methods through the charisma of their personalities. Both disciples and clients have responded to the work largely as an article of faith, and on the basis of anecdotal reports of patients who have made remarkable improvements. Future testing in organized clinical trials may elucidate whether or not these new therapies are significant improvements over conventional allopathic physical therapy.

In conclusion, an interesting contradiction has occurred in medical care over the last decade. On the one hand allopathy has become increasingly scientific in its approach to both patients and methods of treatment. Public health experts and medical practitioners demand proof of the effectiveness of treatments, refusing to accept new advances as an article of faith. Criticisms of coronary care units, new cancer treatments and concern over adverse drug reactions point to this trend. Both the lay and professional public are increasingly skeptical of innovation.

Yet at the same time a significant segment of the population is fleeing from the demand for proof. Perhaps they are saying that proof obscures the purpose of medicine: to relieve pain, cure illness and promote personal growth. Since many of the new therapies have grown in popularity without the underpinnings of proof, these people seem to be saying that faith, empathy and "hands-on" contact may be elements of health care that are valid without the demonstration of effectiveness.

In any case, the contradiction between the allopathic and alternative therapies is more than a curiosity. It is a challenge to both allopathy and the alternative therapies. The likelihood is that the durability and legitimacy of any therapy can come only when proof of its effect is established through its controlled application to many patients, and over a prolonged period. On the other hand, allopathy will have to alter its methods and develop a humanistic side. Furthermore, any form of therapy that is to succeed must meet the emotional as well as the biological needs of its patients.

chapter 5

Acupuncture

In 1971, *New York Times* writer James Reston had his appendix removed while visiting the People's Republic of China. After the surgery, he complained of postoperative nausea and pain, and the hospital staff offered him a unique treatment for his discomfort. They wheeled in an instrument table and inserted some very fine steel needles into his legs, just below the knees. Mr. Reston felt a strange sensation as the attendants twirled the needles, and his nausea quickly diminished. With the wide publicity this experience received, the practice of acupuncture was introduced to an eager American audience. Reston's story was followed by other dramatic accounts of acupuncture's benefits, including surgery using only acupuncture anesthesia and the cure of deafness and paralysis. Acupuncture clinics quickly opened in many American cities, and patients with previously incurable conditions flocked to them, seeking the new miracle treatment from China. The acupuncture boom was on.

In the following 10 years, the miracle cures have been largely discredited, controlled studies have raised serious questions about the value of acupuncture treatment, and acupuncture has been dismissed as a hoax, a placebo and a form of hypnosis. Yet this healing art continues to flourish in the United States. Five states now allow the independent practice of acupuncture by nonphysicians, while 10 more and the District of Columbia allow acupuncturists to practice with the supervision of an M.D. Unfortunately, the public and many professionals are confused and misinformed about acupuncture, partially because of the competing disclaimers made by the allopathic medical establishment on one side and the proponents of acupuncture on the other.

The Heterogeneity of Acupuncture

Acupuncture has been traditionally practiced by the insertion of very fine needles into specific body points that are believed to influence the functioning of the internal organs, the mind and the general state of body energy. The needles are usually made of stainless steel, although some traditional practitioners use gold and silver ones. The insertions are made into the layer of muscle that lies below the skin surface. The depth of insertion varies widely, depending on the amount of fatty tissue in the area of treatment.

Once the needles are in place they are usually left for 15 to 20 minutes, although this too may vary with the philosophy of the practitioner. They may be stimulated manually by periodic hand twirling, or continuously by electrical stimulation. The use of electric current applied directly to the needle is called electro-acupuncture. It is a new technique, but has become standard practice for the majority of acupuncturists in the West. Electro-acupuncture is the technique most often used when acupuncture is studied in clinical trials.

The exact number and location of the acupuncture points used in therapy is a matter of dispute among the different schools and styles of practice. The traditional Chinese method uses, for the most part, points developed by the ancient Chinese acupuncturists. These points have been recorded in textbooks that date to hundreds of years before the birth of Christ. They represent an empirical tradition in Oriental healing, and are probably the earliest medical texts known.

Other practitioners use the traditional points as a foundation, but add newer points discovered in modern China, Japan, Korea and the West. There are some who treat all problems with points located on the ear, and others who have abandoned all the traditional points. These last-named practitioners choose locations based solely on the principles of modern neuroanatomy, or on the basis of electronic measurements made with new instruments. There are even acupuncturists who no longer use needles at all, instead substituting electronic and ultrasonic stimulation applied directly to the skin surface, without penetrating the skin.

The newest area in acupuncture practice focuses on using the traditional Oriental energy-balancing concepts, with scientific measurements obtained with modern electronic instruments. In this model, the flow of body energy (Chi) is redirected to provide internal harmony and health. Practitioners in Japan and Germany have developed new electronic systems, which record physiological changes in the skin surface, and which purportedly indicate potential treatment points. This is a major departure from traditional practice, which uses only the points mapped out over thousands of years of observation. These new practitioners also make their initial diagnoses with the new instruments, shunning the traditional diagnosis, which employs observations of the pulse at the wrist and of the tongue, breath, and skin, as well as other empirical evidence.

One of the new instrument-based acupuncture systems has been developed by a German physician, Rheinhold Voll, who claims to be able to detect disease states in the internal organs by measuring electrical changes with a meter that he has developed. Voll says that this is a historic breakthrough because it provides a scientific method for detecting early disease states, and enables the practitioner to correct imbalances in body energy before they manifest themselves as medical disorders.

Another new method of acupuncture uses low-intensity electrical stimulation applied with electrodes at both traditional acupuncture points and points discovered by electrical measurement. This needleless acupuncture is being used by physical therapists and athletic trainers to help block pain. It may also aid in tissue healing. Preliminary studies indicate that this technique is better than a placebo in producing long-term pain relief after some muscular injuries.

Although acupuncture with electronic devices is new, and as yet largely unproven in scientific testing, many acupuncturists are turning to it as the best hope for securing a firm scientific foundation for acupuncture. They hope to silence the criticisms of allopathic medicine, which has been skeptical about the empirical basis on which acupuncture rests.

The proponents of the new devices still adhere to the basic concepts of Oriental medicine, which state that the body has energy fields that are changed by acupuncture treatment. Some of these proponents cite the use, by orthopedists, of electrical currents in treating extensive bone fractures as an example of how bioelectric fields may play an important role in the future of medical care. However, at this point, neither the theory nor the use of the new electronic acupuncture devices is based on firm experimental evidence.

The heterogenous philosophy and practice on which it has been based has been one reason for confusion over the effectiveness of acupuncture. Reports claiming to document the success or failure of a particular method must be carefully examined to ascertain the techniques that were used for treatment and diagnosis.

There is also controversy over acupuncture diagnosis. The oldest form of this is pulse diagnosis, in which the acupuncturist evaluates changes in the pulse felt at the wrist (the radial artery). Another type of diagnosis is performed by evaluating specific locations on the ear that relate to specific body areas and internal organs (Oleson, 1980). But while this technique is completely foreign to allopathic diagnosis, a study performed at the Pain Control Unit of the University of California at Los Angeles showed a 75% correlation between such ear diagnoses and diagnoses made by standard allopathic methods. Similar studies of pulse diagnosis, tongue diagnosis and the other techniques used in Oriental medicine have not been done.

Acupuncture Therapy for Pain

The simplest and perhaps most effective use of acupuncture involves the insertion of needles directly into areas of muscle pain, leaving the needles in place until the pain diminishes. Often when the needle is removed a few minutes later, the pain is greatly reduced or vanishes completely. The Chinese call this treating the "a-shih" or "ouch" points. In a manual used for training barefoot doctors in China (who have limited training), the procedure is fully described as an everyday approach to pain.

Actually, the same basic technique was advocated by William Osler, one of the most prominent North American physicians of the early twentieth century. In his famous text, *Principles and Practice of Medicine,* Osler claimed that inserting metal needles into the most painful area was an excellent treatment for low back pain. (Osler, 1909)

This technique was further refined by Dr. Janet Travell of the United States (who later became President Kennedy's physician). In the early 1950's, she found that painful muscles contain *trigger points*—sensitive areas that produce predictable pain responses when pressure is applied to them. Dr. Travell found that the "dry needling" of a trigger point (using a standard hypodermic needle, but without injecting medication) would dispell the pain. In some cases this method cured painful problems of many years' duration.

There is a very high degree of correlation between the trigger points identified by Dr. Travell and the classical acupuncture points developed thousands of years ago in China. Since the only difference between dry needling and acupuncture is the size of the needle (the acupuncture needles are much finer), it may be that both methods work in the same physiological way.

The exact mechanism by which both acupuncture and dry needling work is not fully understood. It is thought that two mechanisms are involved: one affecting the central nervous system and the other the painful muscle itself. One theory holds that chronic pain partly results from repeated bombardment of the brain with pain stimuli, and that the insertion of the acupuncture needle breaks this continuous pain cycle.

The second mechanism of pain relief by acupuncture and dry needling involves the reaction of the muscle to the treatment. The muscle first contracts around the needle and then relaxes dramatically. Since continued muscle tension and poor circulation are basic factors in chronic pain, it may be that needling, by relaxing the muscle, increases blood flow to the muscle and relieves local pressure on the peripheral nerves.

Although it is not known why trigger points work, there is some experimental evidence that they are more effective than placebo. In studies of more than 1,000 patients, Dr. Travell and other researchers found that trigger-point stimulation at the correct location provides significantly more pain relief than either no treatment or needling at an incorrect point. The electrical stimulation of needles at incorrect points has also proven less effective than stimulation at the appropriate points.

Acupuncture, like dry needling, has been studied in the treatment of low back pain. In an experiment done in British Columbia, patients who had been unsuccessfully treated with conventional physiotherapy, exercise and occupational therapy were given dry needling at acupuncture points in the lower back. The group treated in this way reported a reduction in their pain and showed an improved ability to return to work. (Gunn, 1980)

Dry needling of trigger points has also been used in the treatment of headaches. This has been applied most consistently for tension headache, which is thought to partly result from chronic muscle tension in the scalp, neck and shoulders. Here the needles are usually inserted into one or more spots in the back of the neck, top of the shoulder, forehead, or temple, and are left in place for 15 to 20 minutes—although some practitioners now use shorter treatment periods.

There have been no controlled studies supporting the effectiveness of dry needling for headache. However, many allopaths as well as alternative healers believe that tension plays a role in headache, and if it does, dry needling may have a positive function in treating headaches.

Although acupuncture has a role in the treatment of pain, the results are not necessarily consistent for all people. In a study done in a private acupuncture clinic in the Washington, D.C., area, for example, 40% of low back patients found some relief from needling, but only 20% were actually rated as cured. Sixty-five percent had either a recurrence of their chronic symptoms or an acute attack of back pain after the treatment (Coan, 1980). Thus, further study is needed to identify the type of client most likely to benefit from acupuncture treatment.

Arthritis and Bursitis

Acupuncture has also been used for treating the chronic pain of arthritis. Like headache, arthritis is a highly heterogeneous disease that includes osteoarthritis (also called degenerative joint disease), rheumatoid arthritis, gouty arthritis and some less common types. There is little information in the acupuncture literature about which type of arthritis—if any—is best treated with acupuncture.

The simplest acupuncture treatment for arthritis involves inserting the needles into points near the affected joints. If there is muscle tension around the painful joint, this therapy may work by breaking the pain cycle in the muscle, in a manner similar to the effect claimed for trigger points and the direct needling of painful muscles.

Another, recently offered explanation—called the *spinal gate theory*—hypothesizes that the insertion of the acupuncture needle blocks the pain message before it can get to the spinal cord and brain. During the period of relief, conventional physical therapy may be applied to further promote pain relief.

A third possible explanation for the effect of acupuncture in arthritis comes from our newly evolving understanding of brain chemistry. In some studies, acupuncture has been shown to promote the release of *endorphins* in the brain. These neurochemicals, especially beta endorphin, are the most potent pain-relieving substances known (beta endorphin is said to be many times more powerful than opium in relieving pain). Although there is a debate over whether acupuncture increases endorphin release—and if so whether it can do this more effectively than a placebo or hypnosis—a number of independent researchers have published studies showing that acupuncture therapy does release endorphins. It has also been shown that naloxone, a drug which counteracts the effects of opium and morphine, can block the pain-relieving effect of acupuncture. Additional research in this area is thus likely to be extremely helpful in understanding the mechanism of acupuncture in treating pain. (Malizia, 1979; Pomerantz, 1979; Sjolund, 1979; Chung, 1980)

If either the spinal gate or endorphin release concepts are actually valid, they may explain why acupuncture works for a variety of pain disorders. Since both concepts involve general physiological reactions, the type of arthritis or exact positioning of the acupuncture needles may not be essential factors in the relief of the pain.

Tendinitis and bursitis have also been treated with acupuncture. The classical Chinese method involves placing needles in the exact position of the pain, but on the opposite side of the body. In the traditional theory this technique works by drawing "excess energy" away from the inflamed side of the body. Here again some skeptics raise the question whether the pain relief is due to placebo effects. Further study is needed to separate specific effects of needling from the nonspecific placebo effects.

Treating Organ Dysfunction

Traditional Chinese acupuncture has been used for centuries to treat virtually every ailment of the internal organs. This is done by using *formula points* that, over the years, have been found to be useful for a variety of problems. In the case of James Reston's nausea, the needles were inserted below the knee, at a formula point that is used to treat problems of the abdomen and digestive organs. The relief of his nausea may therefore have been due to a generalized action on the digestive system, obtained by stimulating the remote point below the knee.

However, the formula points of traditional acupuncture do not correspond to any modern anatomical mapping of the nervous system or major internal organs of the body, which has raised skepticism among allopaths, who have difficulty explaining the effect of acupuncture at these points.

A possible explanation is based on our understanding of one of the major divisions of the nervous system—the autonomic nervous system—which regulates the body's automatic functions (such as digestion, breathing and the heart rate). The autonomic nervous system actually consists of two systems—the parasympathetic nervous system, which produces a lowered heart rate and blood pressure, and promotes digestion; and the sympathetic system, which speeds up the heart rate, raises the blood pressure and slows digestion.

In James Reston's case, stimulation of the formula point below the knee may have produced a generalized stimulation of the sympathetic nervous system, which would have decreased the activity of his digestive system and reduced his nausea.

There is growing experimental evidence to support this theory. Acupuncture has been shown to alter bowel function in experimental animals, and electro-acupuncture has been used to help women with urinary incontinence. Both systems are influenced by the autonomic nervous system (Kubista, 1976). A study at the Hawaii School of Medicine showed that electro-acupuncture at various formula points was helpful in inducing labor in 78% of women with delayed labor. It was also useful for treating 91% of women in premature labor by delaying contractions of the uterus (Tsuei, 1977). The authors of these studies all point to the potential role of acupuncture in stimulating the central nervous system. The next step would be to quantify the production of the specific neurochemicals and show their effects on the internal organs.

Among the internal organ dysfunctions for which acupuncture has been used have been menstrual cramps, asthma, stomach ulcers, irritable bowel syndrome, migraine headache and Raynaud's disease.

Asthma has perhaps been the best studied of these. In one double-blind study at UCLA, acupuncture reduced the airway resistance—the constriction of the air passages that produces wheezing and shortness of breath—in asthmatic patients. In this study, acupuncture was found to be better than placebo (wrong-point) acupuncture or injections of saline (salt water, which has no therapeutic effect). However, it was not as effective as isoproterenol, one of the most potent Western drugs for asthma.

There are few data on the benefit of acupuncture treatment for other common dysfunctions of the internal organs. Some studies have shown it to be beneficial in treating stomach ulcers and menstrual cramps, but these have not controlled for nonspecific placebo effects.

The acupuncture treatment of such habits as overeating, smoking, alcohol, and heroin abuse has usually involved a combination of needles inserted into the external ear surface and small, coiled "ear tacks" that are left in place for days or weeks. The patients simply press on the coiled section of the tack whenever they want to stimulate the ear points being treated. In persons trying to stop smoking, for example, an ear tack will be placed on the "lung" point in the ear, with the subject stimulating the point by pressing on the tack when the desire to smoke arises. If successful, this will relieve the craving for the cigarette.

As with other acupuncture therapies, the exact mechanism by which this system works remains unknown. If it involves generalized stimulation of the central nervous system, it may work through the vagus nerve, which has branches that supply the ear and major internal organs of the chest and abdomen.

Studies of the effectiveness of acupuncture in smoking have produced conflicting results. A Canadian study failed to show that acupuncture was better than placebo acupuncture or self-control in helping people quit smoking. While there was an initial positive placebo effect, all of the treatment groups were equally likely to fall back into the smoking habit after a few weeks of therapy. Both federally funded studies in the United States and tests done in Hong Kong on the control of heroin abuse indicate that acupuncture has a potentially beneficial role, especially for relieving withdrawal symptoms.

Yet it is difficult to say whether acupuncture has a specific role in controlling substance abuse. It may work merely as a simple "reminder" type of therapy; pulling on an ear tack may function like a string tied to one's finger as a reminder not to smoke. Alternatively, the expectation that the therapy will work, coupled with the positive reinforcement of the acupuncturist who administers the treatment, may exert a placebo effect. On the other hand, the treatment may have effects related to stimulation of the central nervous system. Habit control remains a new and relatively untested use of acupuncture.

Finally, although there is no evidence documenting the effect of acupuncture in mental illness, anxiety and insomnia, it is a form of treatment that is increasingly being applied to these areas. The Chinese have used acupuncture as an adjunct to conventional psychiatric medication, and preliminary work in the United States indicates that acupuncture may have a role in treating insomnia and anxiety. This would be another application of the effect of acupuncture on the nervous system.

Maintaining and Restoring Body Harmony

Although the primary use of acupuncture in the West has probably been for the treatment of pain and organ dysfunction, Chinese acupuncturists perceive this approach as fairly primitive. For these healers the true goal is to cure illness by restoring proper balance in the flow of body energy and to prevent illness by maintaining that balance. To the traditional Oriental practitioner disease is seen as an imbalance in the flow of life energy, or Chi; and the healing techniques of meditation, exercise, herbs and acupuncture all work together to correct disarray in the circulation of Chi.

Traditional acupuncturists use pulse diagnosis, tongue diagnosis, voice quality, body odor and food preference to evaluate the basic state of the body's energy. On the basis of these observations different herbs and acupuncture points are chosen to produce a shift in the circulation of Chi. These treatments are not designed to relieve the symptoms of illness or cure disease; they are instead aimed at restoring the body to maximal function.

Chi is maintained through a balance of two basic forces: Yin and Yang, found in both the body and mind. There is a corollary between Yin and the parasympathetic nervous system, since Yin emphasizes the passive functions of digestion and secretion. Yang, on the other hand, is more like the sympathetic nervous system which operates during the "fight or flight" reaction. Balancing Yin and Yang therefore not only makes the individual feel better, but also promotes resistance to physical and psychological illness.

This characteristic of acupuncture is appealing to holists and other alternative healers, who consider the prevention of illness and the maintenance of optimal mind and body function as the highest of all therapeutic goals. Not surprisingly, traditional Oriental medicine was instantly appealing to the proponents of alternative healing. By and large, these practitioners were already involved in Oriental philosophy during the late 1960's, and accepted the empirical assumptions of Eastern religion.

However, there has been no way to effectively test the Chi hypothesis. Its very nature baffles the modern view of illness, and we have no way to measure Chi. The Western biological concept of homeostasis posits that all organisms have a tendency to restore themselves to biological equilibrium, but this too is only theory. So far, allopathy regards the Chi concept as an article of faith, accepted by both the practitioners and clients of traditional Oriental medicine.

The Dangers of Acupuncture

When acupuncture first exploded into the Western healing arts, many persons were concerned that the insertion of needles by nonphysician practitioners would produce dangerous side effects and adverse reactions. The Texas State Board of Medical Examiners, for instance, prohibited nonphysician acupuncturists from practicing, claiming that this would reduce the likelihood of dangerous complications from acupuncture treatment. The Board also stated that M.D. practitioners would be more likely to recognize the complications of acupuncture treatment, and would be able to treat them more promptly and effectively than nonphysician practitioners. Other observors claimed that unsterilized needles would spread a variety of infections, especially potentially serious hepatitis.

However, there is little evidence to support these contentions. Acupuncture is safe when employed by trained practitioners, including both physician and nonphysician healers. At the UCLA pain clinic, over 18,000 acupuncture treatments have been studied, with the principal side effect or adverse reaction being bruising. Naturally, acupuncture needles should be sterilized after use to prevent the transmission of infectious disease. But to date there have been no recorded outbreaks of hepatitis or other infections from acupuncture treatment.

Another criticism of acupuncture has been its potential for puncturing internal organs through faulty needle placement. One case of a collapsed lung from needling was reported by Dr. Arthur Taub, professor of anesthesiology at Yale University, in *The Health Robbers* (Barrett and Knight, 1976). Other reports of injury have involved puncture of the liver, spleen, bladder, kidneys and pregnant uterus. There has been at least one report of death due to needle puncture of the heart.

Some of these incidents have apparently involved physician acupuncturists who were poorly trained in point location. Therefore, M.D. status does not insure the safety of acupuncture. One should be suspicious of the insertion of any long needle, or penetration deeper than just below the skin surface. Any needle insertion on the trunk should be superficial. Moreover, most acupuncture should be performed on the limbs or ear, far away from the vital organs.

Acupuncture and Placebo

Many techniques can improve one's sense of overall well-being and catalyze the placebo response. The immense publicity that acupuncture enjoyed during its introduction into the West probably helped it in these respects. Like meditation, exercise, massage, psychotherapy and faith (religion), acupuncture has important nonspecific effects, but these are not readily amenable to accurate scientific testing. There is, however, a growing body of evidence to suggest that acupuncture is more than a placebo form of therapy. Future scientific studies should help us document the specific healing properties and limits to acupuncture therapy.

chapter 6

The Drug Therapies

The explosive proliferation of "natural" drug therapies —vitamins, herbs, and homeopathic remedies—is a symptom of the misuse of drugs throughout Western society. In the United States there are more than one billion prescriptions filled each year, at a cost of *$11.3 billion.* At least one out of eight of these is for a drug that is either unnecessary or ineffective. The use and abuse of nonprescription medicines occurs on an even larger scale.

We have become a society of pill takers. For many people, any small pain, tension, or discomfort requires a medicinal nostrum. The United States Department of Commerce estimates that 15.9 million men and 25.8 million women take more than one aspirin a week. Even more disturbing is that 3.7 million men and 6.7 million women take more than one sleeping pill each week. Moreover, in 1978 there were 68 million prescriptions written for minor tranquilizers, over half of which were for Valium[T]. This despite the fact that both physicians and the general public know that these medications often cover up emotional problems that should not be treated in this fashion. These drugs are also potentially addicting. They may produce emotional and sleep disturbances that aggravate already existing psychological problems, and may damage the internal organs of the body. When taken with alcohol, they can be fatal. In 1978 there were 22,000 admissions to emergency rooms because of tranquilizer misuse.

Furthermore, the problem of drug reliance is increasing in its severity. In 1975 vitamin sales accounted for $452 million, cough and cold preparations sold for $735 million, and analgesics for $719 million. By 1980 vitamins had increased in sales to $621 million, cough and cold preparations to $968 million and analgesics to $1.129 billion. We seem to have lost faith in our own bodily fortitude, and in the idea that in the normal process of living the body heals itself of most ailments.

The medical and pharmaceutical industry is largely to blame for this staggering drug misuse. The Health Research Group, founded by Ralph Nader, lists over 600 regularly prescribed medications that "are not considered effective by the government's own standards." The Group estimates that in 1979 the cost to buyers of these unproven remedies was more than $1 billion. Dr. Paul Stolley, Professor of Medicine at the University of Pennsylvania, wrote in the Preface to *Pills That Don't Work:*

> An often neglected aspect of a physician's training and continued education concerns the rational use of drugs. The task of updating physicians after graduation has been largely assumed by the drug manufacturers themselves through conferences, journals, promotional materials and visits to physicians by drug company sales representatives. The information provided by drug manufacturers, while subject to Food and Drug Administration scrutiny and regulation, does not necessarily convey the attitudes of skepticism, objectivity, [and] concern with consumer costs or the choices of alternatives, including *no* drug therapy. (Wolfe, 1980)

The allopathic health industry is guilty of enormous abuses in prescribing. What your doctor does not know about drugs may promote expensive, unnecessary and potentially dangerous drug taking. For instance, 10 to 20% of hospital patients have some adverse drug reaction to a medicine prescribed by their physician. Usually this is a mild reaction such as gastrointestinal upset, but occasionally it may be fatal. And given the fact that literally *millions* of prescriptions are written each year for hospital patients, the number of serious and fatal reactions is significant. Further, between 2 and 5% of outpatient prescriptions produce an adverse reaction. Again, this figure may appear small, but actually looms incredibly large when multiplied by the millions of outpatient prescriptions written annually.

Consumers must be skeptical and cautious about taking any medications, whether promoted by the allopathic profession or by an alternative healer. The Health Research Group makes this point:

> Even though the FDA requires labeling and advertising for many of these drugs [drugs which have not been proven effective in rigorous tests] to include a small box indicating

> the drugs lack evidence of effectiveness, many doctors pay as much attention to these little boxes as do smokers to the Surgeon General's warning box on cigarettes. Besides, many doctors think that if they judge a drug to work, even if scientific studies show it doesn't, they have the right to prescribe it. Early in the 1950's, DES [diethylstilbesterol] was shown in published, well controlled studies not to protect women from miscarriage. Nevertheless, *after* this time, it was prescribed to prevent miscarriages in millions of women because some doctors "believed" the drug worked. Each had seen a woman with a miscarriage in a previous pregnancy take DES and avoid a miscarriage during a subsequent pregnancy. Blinded to the notion that it was not DES but just the natural variation from one pregnancy to the next [that prevented such miscarriage], doctors rejected scientific studies in deference to their own personal "experience" and therefore exposed millions of mothers, sons and daughters to DES, the effects of which have included cancer, birth defects, and problems with pregnancies. (Wolfe, 1980)

These observations apply equally to the alternative drug therapies. Friends, practitioners and lay healers often suggest remedies that have never been demonstrated to be either safe or effective. They do this on the basis of personal experience or hearsay that has nothing to do with scientific proof of effectiveness. In some cases, the positive experience with these "natural" remedies is a result of the placebo effect or the normal tendency for the body to heal itself of most medical illnesses.

There is a common misconception among many people that because something is labeled as "natural" it is safe. Drugs such as herbs are often poorly packaged, incorrectly labeled, contaminated with illegally added prescription drugs, or in the case of laetrile (amygdalin)—which contains cyanide—highly toxic. In short, the consumer interest in alternative drug therapies is no more rational than the misuse of conventional pharmaceuticals. Yet it is escalating at an incredible rate. In 1978 laetrile sales came to more than $1 billion, not including fees for the injection and oral administration of laetrile, or for enzymes, vitamins and other nutritional supplements associated with laetrile therapy.

People have turned to the alternative drug therapies for a variety of reasons. There is confusion about and frustration with conventional allopathic medicines, which are often considered unnecessarily expensive and potentially dangerous. In addition, many people want to be able to diagnose and treat some of their own illnesses, especially those that they feel are simple or minor. Often patients resent having to go to a physician for a prescription when they know the cause of their problem and what they need to treat it. They resent that many common medications such as antibiotics and minor pain killers are controlled drugs, apparently kept that way to increase doctors' incomes.

Nevertheless, there is little that is safe or efficacious about alternative drug therapy. In contrast to the nondrug therapies such as biofeedback, acupuncture, meditation, Rolfing, massage, and chiropractic, it can be very dangerous.

In deciding to take any medicine one must always weigh the risks and rewards. In scientific circles this is often called the risk/reward ratio. If a medication has not been shown to be effective, the reward is zero and the risk/reward ratio is completely unacceptable, since any quotient with zero as the denominator produces infinity. Even a medication with a small risk is pointless if its reward may be nil. Since few, if any, of the alternative drug therapies have been proven in any rigorous way to have rewards, their risk/reward ratios are, until proven otherwise, unacceptable.

Fortunately, most people rely on alternative drug therapies for minor and self-limited problems. In a study of 400 health-food-store patrons in Stockholm, Sweden, the majority of users were healthy people. They used vitamin, mineral, cereal and herbal preparations for preventive care, and not to treat active medical problems. The remaining patrons, who were seeking drugs for ongoing medical problems, were treating minor conditions like constipation, viral illnesses (which get better on their own), nervous conditions and arthritis.

The information on which these patrons based their choice of a medicinal product usually came from the health-food-store owner, friends, or articles in the popular press. Consumers pointed out that the store owner was more service oriented than the conventional pharmacist, and enjoyed more personalized contact with the patrons.

There may be a lesson in this for both the pharmacist and physician. People want a more personal relationship with their healers, and seek it in the alternative healing modalities. As pharmacists have begun vending everything from beach apparel to school supplies, their customers have increasingly sought drug therapies dispensed by empathetic and interested health-food-store owners and alternative healers. The flight from conventional medicine is likely to continue as long as the physician and pharmacist continue their flight from the consumer.

Herbal Medicine

Traditional herbal medicine is still used to treat 75 to 80% of the world's population. In many developing countries traditional herbal remedies are compatible with indigenous cultures, are locally available, and are far less expensive than drugs produced in the advanced industrialized nations. Often these underdeveloped nations have severe balance-of-payment problems, and purchasing medicines from abroad represents an unfortunate choice between drugs and other necessities such as food, energy or needed technology.

Nature contains an enormous quantity of potentially therapeutic botanicals. The World Health Organization, the governments of many Eastern European countries, the Soviet Union, China, Japan and to a lesser extent several cancer research programs in the United States all support scientific investigation into naturally occurring medicinal plants. Thirty percent of the pharmaceuticals used in developed nations are derived in whole or part from plant sources. Reserpine, for instance, which is made from a plant, is an antihypertensive medication that has been in widespread use for 30 years. Its sales are more than $30 million annually. Yet there are other plants such as *Eucommia,* hellebore, olive (*Olea europea*) and geranium whose extracts also have blood-pressure-lowering properties. Work on all of these botanicals, however, is still only in the research stage. In some cases they are too toxic for human consumption or unsuitable for general use for other reasons.

Testing botanicals for medical use is a long process. Initially a preparation must be isolated and given to laboratory animals. If these tests demonstrate that the preparation is safe and effective, the next step is to perform a series of clinical trials in humans, testing for toxicity and therapeutic efficacy in small numbers of volunteer subjects. If these initial studies show promise, enlarged studies can be done, comparing the natural remedy to both placebo and a pharmaceutical of known efficacy. With time and testing these studies can demonstrate who is most likely to benefit from a new drug, the proper dose of the drug, and any potentially harmful side effects. Often this last area is the one that takes the most time to reveal: adverse drug reactions and complications of therapy can occur years after the administration of a drug. In short, the demonstration that a "natural" remedy is safe and effective is a slow and painstaking process.

Such a demonstration has been undertaken in India with an herbal mixture known as LIV 52. This remedy has been used for a variety of purposes by traditional Indian healers, and specifically in the treatment of infectious hepatitis, which is epidemic in India. After laboratory tests in animals showed that LIV 52 could afford some protection from liver cancer, small scale testing was tried in humans. When used in both children and adults, LIV 52 appeared to be somewhat useful for reducing the symptoms of hepatitis and in promoting a more rapid recovery from the disease.

But such rational scientific investigation into the usefulness of plant substances bears little or no relationship to the indiscriminate and often foolhardy use of these substances by "natural" drug enthusiasts in the Western nations. Dr. G. B. Martini-Bettólo pointed this out in the 1980 *Journal of Ethnopharmacology:*

> Moreover, we must recognize that in many industrialized countries there is a parallel market [to that of allopathy] of [using] not always sound, plant products [herbalism], especially in the last years on the wave of naturism and ecology. (Martini-Bettólo, 1980)

Both physicians and nonphysicians have been guilty of promoting often dangerous "natural" therapies. For instance, Dr. John Eiselle, the medical examiner of King County, Washington, reported the case of a 46-year-old woman who had previously been diagnosed as having colitis and gall-bladder disease, and at her physician's suggestion began a dietary program of fresh fruits and juices supplemented with nutritional preparations. Shortly before her death she began to have abdominal pain, and was told to start regular coffee enemas. She administered 10 to 12 of these treatments to herself on the first night, and continued with this therapy for the next few days. She eventually became depleted of the salts (electrolytes) needed to maintain normal body chemistry, had a grand mal seizure, was taken to the hospital in a coma, and died despite efforts to restore her internal chemical balance.

This story is not the only one of death or serious illness produced by abuses of "natural" remedies. In 1980, for instance, a 54-year-old North Carolina construction worker was admitted to the hospital with arsenic poisoning caused by drinking tea made from "yellow root" *(Xanthorrhiza sp.)* picked near his home. The plant was evidently contaminated by water and soil pollutants produced in nearby industrial plants. Several children have died from eating the berries of the pokeweed plant (also known as the inkbury), and in 1977 two people died who had ingested a plant they thought was comfrey *(Symphytum),* but which, in fact, was foxglove. This produced a fatal overdose of digitalis.

The April 1979 issue of the *Medical Letter on Drugs and Therapeutics* lists more than 30 potentially toxic plants used medicinally by humans. Some, like goldenrod, marigold and yarrow, produce only minor allergic reactions. Licorice root, however, can produce cardiac toxicity, and pennyroyal may induce spontaneous abortion (miscarriage) as well as causing liver and kidney damage. Indian tobacco *(lobelia)* is effective for inducing vomiting, but when taken in an overdose is a potent central nervous system stimulant that can produce paralysis, coma and death. Burdock root contains an anticholinergic drug that causes blurred vision, dilated pupils, a dry mouth and other nervous system disorders.

Furthermore, improperly packaged herbal preparations may contain potentially carcinogenic fungi called aflatoxins, and in some preparations, pathologic bacteria such as *Salmonella* have been found. In short, just because a product is packaged as "natural" does not mean that it is fit for human consumption.

Another potential danger of herbal remedies is that there is no guarantee that the product has been properly collected or labeled. Since the herbs in these remedies are often picked by people with little or no knowledge of botanicals, it is possible to purchase toxic plants that the vendor thinks are safe. It is also hard to tell one dried herb from another. And health-food-store proprietors are rarely (if ever) accountable for the safety of the products they sell. Nor are herbal medicines currently regulated as either food or drug. In short, there is no control of the product, its collection, packaging, or sale.

Dr. Ryan Huxtable of the University of Arizona investigated the use of "Gordoloba Tea" which had been implicated in the death of a 2-month-old Mexican-American child. He found that consumers were purchasing a potentially toxic plant known as thread-leaf groundsel (also known as woolly groundsel). This plant contains potentially lethal chemicals called pyrrolizidines. The plant had been packaged in a popcorn wrapper as a cough remedy. Evidently Mexican-Americans who purchased the tea were under the impression that it was the same as a remedy they used in Mexico under the same name. But the plant remedy they were familiar with, *Gnaphalium macounii*—which has been used by traditional healers called curenderos—does not contain pyrrolizidines. This potentially dangerous herbal remedy was also sold in other parts of the country under a variety of names, including Punchon, Mullein, Tobaco Cimarron and Manzanilla de Rio.

There is also considerable potential danger involved in purchasing herbal or "natural" remedies produced outside the United States. There have been many accounts of poisoning, some fatal, from these products. In a University of California study of 133 ginseng users (mostly taking imported products) over a 2-year period, many individuals showed intermittent symptoms of skin eruption, appetite suppression, edema, alterations in normal blood pressure, euphoria and depression. The researchers found that the ginseng was sometimes contaminated with steroids, estrogens and other potentially toxic drugs. Another study found ginseng to contain scopolomine (a powerful central nervous system medication authorized only for use as an anesthetic during surgical procedures), and snake root, which contains reserpine (a central nervous system depressant).

Similarly, a few cases of agranulocytosis, a potentially fatal disease of the bone marrow, have been associated with the use of Chuei-Fong-Tou-Geuwan, an herbal preparation sold for the treatment of arthritis. Among the contaminants found in this remedy have been steroids (dexamethasone), nonsteroidal antiinflammatory agents (indomethacin, phenylbutasone), analgesics (phenacetin, which may produce kidney damage), mercuric sulfide (a toxic heavy metal) and aminopyrene (illegal in the United States because it is known to produce agranulocytosis). (Ries, 1975)

In 1981 the *British Medical Journal* reported the case of

a 49-year-old housewife who was admitted to the hospital complaining of nausea, malaise and aching pains in her abdomen. Blood tests revealed that she had hepatitis, apparently contracted from an herbal pill containing a number of substances including mistletoe. Yet while mistletoe is known to be toxic, a pharmacy in Portsmouth, England, reportedly sold 30,000 capsules of this remedy a week. It was promoted for a variety of disorders, including epilepsy, asthma, and infertility, and as an aphrodisiac. It has never been demonstrated to be effective for any of these conditions. (Harvey, 1981)

Other foreign preparations have also been associated with serious toxicity. A 59-year-old woman was admitted to a San Francisco-area hospital with symptoms of insomnia, pain in her knees and breasts, irritability, paranoia, anemia and constipation. Under treatment by a local herbalist and acupuncturist for arthritis, she had been given an herbal preparation that contained lead, which had produced lead poisoning. When questioned by the authorities, the healer said that he had had no idea that the client was suffering from lead poisoning or that the herbal preparation contained lead. (Lightfoote, 1977)

In summary, there are a number of reasons why an herbal or "natural" remedy may not be safe:

1. The product may have faulty packaging and contain fungal or bacterial contaminants capable of producing infection, cancer or a drug reaction.
2. The substance may have been collected improperly, so that the material in the package is not what it is purported to be.
3. The product may contain toxic drugs or chemicals that have been added to the herbal product.

4. There is no standardization of potency. Brewing the remedy as a tea, adding it to blenderized drinks or food, taking it as a pill, or using it in the form of an enema, may produce a wide variability in the amount of the substance ingested.

Consumers should be aware that both lay healers and allopaths have little or no formal training in the use of herbal remedies. Dr. Vicenzo Picci of the Institute of Botanical Pharmacology of the University of Sassari, Italy, pointed this out in the *Journal of Ethnopharmacology:*

> [T]he use of medicinal species in herbalistic practice is not based on adequate knowledge of the problem by most medical practitioners. In the medical facilities very little knowledge is acquired regarding medicinal plants, and the information available is often inaccurate; also, the plant materials obtained are not always genuine, and are not sufficiently standardized. (Picci, 1980)

Unfortunately many consumers and healers have erroneously turned to natural remedies because they intuitively feel that they must be safe. In doing so they are basing their decision more on the dangers they perceive to be inherent in modern pharmaceuticals than on the proven safety of herbal or natural substances. For some this has meant jumping from the frying pan and into the fire.

Megadose Vitamins, "Orthomolecular" and Nutritional Therapy

Public interest in and consumption of vitamin, mineral and nutritional therapies currently exceeds that for all other forms of alternative medicine. More than half a billion dollars is spent annually on vitamin preparations. Laetrile, although technically not a vitamin, has been touted as vitamin B_{17}, and itself accounts for more than $1 billion in sales and fees. There are no reliable figures on the sales of digestive enzymes, mineral supplements, protein mixtures, and other such preparations, but these products undoubtedly account for added millions.

More misconceptions exist about the use of vitamins than about any other form of alternative therapy. For instance, in a study done in the early 1970's by the FDA, 71% of the general public (and 75% of health-food-store patrons) erroneously believed that the symptoms of fatigue and "feeling run down" were likely to be a result of vitamin or mineral deficiency. This belief is communicated by those alternative healers who support "orthomolecular medicine," despite the lack of studies demonstrating that vitamin deficiency produces these symptoms, or that vitamin supplementation will correct them (except in rare diseases such as megaloblastic anemia, which will be discussed later).

The FDA found that consumers also held other false notions about the role of vitamins in human nutrition. Sixty-seven percent of the general public (and 73% of health-food enthusiasts) felt that older people had different vitamin requirements than younger people. Thirty-seven percent of health-food enthusiasts felt that cancer and arthritis were partially caused by vitamin deficiencies. Twenty-three percent felt that they could protect themselves from illness by adding extra vitamins to their diet. A staggering 86% believed that "natural" vitamins were better and more useful to the body than synthetically produced ones. Yet although each one of these notions is held by vast numbers of people, they are all false.

It is not the average consumer who is to blame for having these misconceptions; they are spread by misleading stories in the popular press and by promotional advertising, because vitamins are big business. Unfortunately, such misconceptions are exceedingly costly in terms of health dollars and misleading in terms of promoting good health and nutrition habits, and in certain cases have promoted toxic and fatal misuse of these nutritional substitutes.

As an example of how false and misleading information about vitamins (and nutrition generally) is spread, the March 13, 1978, *New York Magazine* carried a cover story declaring vitamin B_{15} (pangamic acid) to be a potential cure "for everything short of a transit strike." Within 2 weeks virtually every available bottle in the New York area had been sold. But pangamic acid is not a vitamin, not useful for a single medical problem and not even an identifiable chemical substance—and it is potentially toxic. It is banned for sale in Canada because it is useless and possibly harmful, and has been removed from the *Merck Index* of chemical substances because it is highly heterogeneous. In short, there is no such thing as vitamin B_{15}, and what is sold as such may be harmful, not beneficial, for one's health. Few people, in fact, know what a vitamin is, or what it does when it enters the human body.

The Function of Vitamins

Thirteen vitamins are necessary to maintain normal human function. Four of these—vitamins, A, D, E and K, are fat soluble—while the eight B-complex vitamins (thiamin, riboflavin, niacin, B_6, pantothenic acid, B_{12}, biotin, folic acid) and ascorbic acid (vitamin C) are water soluble. All are organic chemicals that the body does not make in sufficient quantities to maintain normal metabolism. Therefore, they must be ingested in the form of food.

Vitamins function as coenzymes that play an essential role in regulating the body's metabolism. When they are ingested, they pass from the digestive tract into the blood stream. From there they must enter the cells of the body and join with a protein (called an apoenzyme) to form an active protein-enzyme complex called a holoenzyme. Vitamins are not nutritionally active by themselves; they perform their regulatory function only when connected to the apoenzyme and form a holoenzyme. Moreover, vitamins are not useful as a source of energy. We do not "burn" vitamins for this purpose as we do fat, protein and carbohydrate.

Another common misperception is that taking *more* vitamins than the daily minimum suggested by nutritionists promotes better health. This is false for a number of reasons. First, because vitamins act only as coenzymes attached to an apoenzyme, the amount of a vitamin that is needed is limited by the amount of apoenzyme present in the cell—which is regulated by the metabolic needs of the body. Without an added amount of apoenzyme, an added amount of vitamin has no biological function. Flooding the cell with extra vitamins is therefore usually wasteful. Second, in some cases, an amount of vitamin greater than the minimum needed to maintain healthy cell regulation can be toxic.

Many consumers also believe that the food purchased in most supermarkets has had its vitamins altered or removed during growth, harvesting or packaging. But while this may be true of some canned products, it does not lead to vitamin deficiency. Many criticisms of the typical American diet can be made, including its excessive content of fat, sugar, salt and refined carbohydrates; but there is no evidence of vitamin deficiency in normal persons who eat an average diet. In fact, few medical practitioners have ever seen a case of vitamin deficiency not associated with alcoholism or with a psychological illness in which the patient does not eat enough food. Moreover, the decline in the incidence of tuberculosis, diphtheria and other infectious disease is largely the result of improved nutrition and hygiene rather than of the development of antibiotics or vaccination. Thus, while poor diet is a serious medical problem in America and other Western nations, it is because we have too much food, and eat the wrong types of foods, rather than because of vitamin deficiency.

A third fallacy is that because vitamins are "natural," taking large amounts of them is harmless. In the case of the water-soluble B vitamins and vitamin C, excessive doses usually produce only minor symptoms such as gastrointestinal upset, headache, or inflammation of the urinary tract. However, taking large doses of the fat-soluble vitamins, particularly vitamins A and D, is not safe. These chemicals are stored in the fat cells of the body, and their prolonged overingestion can produce kidney, liver, bone and eye damage. As we shall later see, amygdalin (laetrile)—often sold as vitamin B_{17}, although it is not a vitamin—is extremely toxic. It contains cyanide and has caused death in at least 16 people. In African countries, where laetriles are found in some of the indigenous foods (such as in the cassava consumed by Nigerians), they have been for years known to produce serious neurological disease.

Another popular misconception is that for some reason nutritionists and the government conspire to downplay the amount of vitamins necessary for good health. Some health faddists also claim that little is actually known about vitamins, and that new vitamins are likely to be discovered with future research.

In fact, vitamins are among the better understood components of human nutrition. The last vitamin to be discovered was vitamin B_{12}, isolated in 1948. No new vitamins have since been uncovered despite 30 years of active research. Moreover, the minimum daily requirement of vitamins has been established on the *high side,* i.e., with an added safety factor, to insure that vitamin deficiencies do not occur in the general public. In the last few years the minimum daily requirement has even been *reduced,* as nutritionists have realized that it was initially set too high in order to avoid deficiency states in the general public. In fact, such vitamin-deficiency diseases as scurvy, pellagra, beri beri and rickets are generally unheard of in the general American population. Few physicians have ever seen any cases of these disorders other than those associated with severe malnutrition, alcoholism, or severe psychological disease.

Another argument against the notion that little is known about vitamins or the minimum amount of vitamins needed to maintain normal metabolism is that hospital patients are now kept alive solely on synthetic intravenous diets, in which the necessary vitamin content has been meticulously established. These patients show normal metabolic function, without any apparent evidence of vitamin deficiency.

Finally, the concept of "vitamin deficiency" has been abused and misused by the media and faddists to promote sales of unnecessary vitamin supplements. A vitamin deficiency is an illness that produces definite clinical symptoms, which can be reversed by adding the appropriate vitamin(s) to the diet. The symptoms of "fatigue," malaise, irritability and lack of energy are not commonly associated with rickets, scurvy and pellagra for example. Controlled clinical experiments have never shown that vitamin supplementation reverses these somewhat vague symptoms. People who feel more alive and energized when taking vitamins are probably demonstrating a positive psychological placebo effect due to their own expectations of benefit. They start out believing that vitamins will restore their energy and fulfill their own prophecies.

There are only a few medical indications for the use of vitamin supplements. One instance is when someone has to take a prescription medication that depletes or antagonizes the function of a vitamin (such as isoniazid for tuberculosis, or methotrexate and hexamethylmelamine, which are used in some types of cancer chemotherapy). Other cases are due to uncommon genetic errors of metabolism (such as homocystinuria and Hartnup's disease). A third instance is when illness or surgery injure the intestinal tract and interfere with the transport of vitamins from the gut into the blood stream. In these cases a vitamin is given as a medicine, for the treatment of a specific deficiency state. Unfortunately, even large doses of vitamins may not be successful in some of these problems.

The American Society for Clinical Nutrition, of the American Dietetic Association, is concerned that the megavitamin craze not only represents a movement toward self-diagnosis and self-dosing, but that it is largely economically wasteful. The Society points out that the large sums of money spent on vitamin supplements could be better spent on wholesome food, particularly by the faddist who buys unnecessarily expensive "natural" vitamins in health-food stores, believing that they are in some way different or better than those purchased in the supermarket. Recognizing that otherwise healthy people need only a balanced diet that contains the appropriate energy stores, plus the recommended amount of daily vitamins and minerals, the Society, in 1978, stated that:

> The National Nutrition Consortium is concerned about people who take large amounts of vitamins. This practice seems to be based on a sincere interest in nutrition and health, but, ironically, it is not a wise practice in terms of either nutrition or health. . . .
>
> The Consortium's concern arises because some people seem to think that if a small amount of a vitamin is good for you, then a large amount must be better. *This assumption is false.* There are important reasons why large amounts of vitamins should not be taken.
>
> The strongest reason is that large doses of certain vitamins, particularly A and D, are known to be dangerous. Extremely large amounts may cause headaches, blurred vision, damage to the nervous system, and other bad effects. Amounts too small to cause noticeable harm, but still well in excess of the RDA, may interfere with the normal body processes such as nerve transmission, body protein formation, hormone action, or blood circulation. These changes are perhaps even of greater concern because they generally occur without their hazards being observed by the [person taking the vitamin], much less corrected by a doctor. (National Nutrition Consortium, 1978)

The immense health-food and alternative healing interest in vitamin supplementation is often stated as a political and philosophical criticism of the environment, the mass production of food or the stresses present in modern living.

While these criticisms are valid in the economic, social and political forum, they are not valid medically.

Megadose C and Other Vitamins

Probably the most abused and misunderstood vitamin is vitamin C (ascorbic acid). Thousands, if not millions, of people take vitamin C for an incredible diversity of ills, ranging from the common cold to cancer. The current public interest in vitamin C was partly catalyzed by Nobel Laureate Dr. Linus Pauling, who began extolling the potential virtues of vitamin C more than a decade ago. He argued that many people needed several grams of ascorbic acid daily, and that the nutritional community had vastly underestimated the appropriate daily need for optimal health. Pauling's promotion of it encouraged people to increase their daily intake to 10 to 50 times the amount recommended by conventional nutritionists.

Ascorbic acid is somewhat unusual in that very few animals require it as an additive to their diet. Only the primates (including humans), guinea pigs, rainbow trout, and a few other species need it. During evolution, these animals may have had vitamin C available in their natural food sources, and hence were able to survive without a crucial enzyme (3-keto-L-gulonate), which other animal species have, and for which vitamin C is a substitute in metabolic regulation.

Scurvy is still the principal disease caused by vitamin C deficiency. It was the scourge of mariners, who spent long periods aboard ship without fresh fruits and vegetables. The demonstration that fresh citrus fruit could reverse the symptoms of scurvy—which include weakness, pain in the muscles and joints, swollen, bleeding gums, anemia, tooth loss, fever and convulsions—was made in the eighteenth century by Dr. James Lind, in an early clinical trial. Today scurvy is extremely rare because fresh fruits and vegetables are readily available, and because vitamin C is often added to juices and other foods.

Ascorbic acid works in concert with other enzymes in a variety of metabolic roles. In the intestine it aids in transforming iron into a biologically useful form; it is needed for producing collagen (a basic constituent of the body's connective tissues); and may play a role in the immune response. It is presumably for the last reason that some people have sought to use vitamin C for treating the common cold and cancer.

Since Pauling's claim for the usefulness of vitamin C in the common cold, a number of experiments have been performed to test this hypothesis. The largest were done at the University of Toronto during the winters of 1971–72, 1972–73, and 1973–74. The tests were designed to see if ascorbic acid would be effective in either preventing colds or reducing their severity.

The initial study employed 1,000 people, taking 1 gram of vitamin C, compared to a placebo group. Persons who developed colds were instructed to take 4 grams of vitamin C each day for the first 3 days of their illness. The results of the first year's trial indicated that both the vitamin C and placebo groups had an equal frequency of colds, but that the vitamin C group had 30% fewer days of work lost or days spent indoors.

The next year an even larger study was undertaken, to test the first year's results, and to examine the effect of dosage. In this study 3,520 subjects were entered, of whom

2,349 completed the study. There were some problems for both the vitamin C and placebo groups, because the large doses of ascorbic acid that were needed necessitated using large pills that some people found undesirable or hard to swallow. As far as demonstrating that vitamin C prevented colds or influenced their overall severity or duration, the results of this follow-up study were even less positive than the first. When a third study was done the next winter, the positive role of large doses (megadoses) of vitamin C was found to be negligible. It was concluded that if vitamin C had any potential benefit for reducing the severity of colds, it could be obtained by taking 100 to 200 mg per day—about the recommended daily dose. Moreover, there was no evidence that daily megadoses of vitamin C prevented the common cold. In short, there is no solid evidence that supplemental vitamin C is of potential benefit in the common cold. One can easily get the recommended daily requirement from a conventional diet that includes juice, fresh fruit and vegetables.

Megadose vitamin C has also been touted for the prevention and treatment of cancer. Initial reports by Drs. Ewan Cameron and Linus Pauling of their work at a regional hospital in Loch Lomondside, Scotland, indicated that doses of up to 10 grams of vitamin C daily were effective in both extending the survival and improving the symptoms of patients being treated for cancer. Megadose vitamin C has also been used with laetrile for cancer treatment.

No independent studies have ever corroborated the findings of Drs. Cameron and Pauling. The Department of Oncology at the Mayo Clinic reported a trial of patients with advanced cancer who failed to respond to large doses of vitamin C added to their conventional therapy. The Mayo scientists found that vitamin C was not better than placebo for reducing the symptoms of illness, increasing weight gain, improving appetite, increasing activity level, or improving the survival of the patients in the study. Also, there has not been a single controlled study (including the work of Drs. Cameron and Pauling—which has been criticized for lacking adequate controls) showing that large doses of vitamin C prevent cancer.

Dr. Victor Herbert, Director of the Hematology and Nutrition Laboratory at the Bronx Veteran's Administration Hospital in New York City, and an opponent of the alternative vitamin and nutritional industry, commented on the work of Drs. Pauling and Cameron:

> The "many years of experience of Dr. Ewan Cameron with megadoses of vitamin C" is typical anecdotal and testimonial citation, useful in advertising but scientifically worthless. A year ago I visited the regional hospital in Scotland where Dr. Cameron works to speak with him. He happened to be on vacation and I spoke with his executive secretary and a senior nurse on a ward where he puts his patients. It was indicated to me that all his patients are given mega-C, that they usually discontinue it because it makes them nauseated or gives them diarrhea, and that no double-blind controlled studies were then being done to their knowledge. (*Journal of Clinical Nutrition,* January, 1980)

In fact, large doses of vitamin C have been implicated in producing several adverse drug reactions. They can irritate the intestinal tract and produce watery diarrhea, and can cause kidney stones and inflammation of the urinary tract. The latter condition produces a syndrome of pus-like discharge from the urethra, along with burning and pain upon urination. Large doses of ascorbic acid have also been implicated in causing a scurvy-like syndrome that apparently results from the body sensing the overingestion of vitamin C and elaborating substances to destroy it. Moreover, when megadoses of vitamin C are discontinued, the vitamin C level may decrease rapidly, producing a condition that resembles the deficiency state. Additionally, vitamin C in megadose quantities can depress vitamin B_{12} levels in the blood, and in people with sickle cell anemia and glucose-6-phosphate dehydrogenase (G-6-PD) deficiency (two genetically inherited enzyme disorders), large doses of the vitamin may precipitate a hemolytic crisis. (Vitler, 1980)

In conclusion, controlled studies have never demonstrated the use of megadose vitamin C to be beneficial for overall good health, or for the prevention or treatment of illness. There is no reason to take more than the 100 to 200 milligrams per day recommended by nutritionists. This amount can be readily obtained in the diet without purchasing supplemental vitamin C tablets. Dr. Richard Vitler summarized this view in the *Western Journal of Medicine:*

> Ascorbic acid in physiological doses is essential for the normal function of the human body. Occasionally, massive doses may be necessary to compensate for a defective enzyme system, but otherwise megadoses of the vitamin for the prevention of colds, healing of wounds and therapy of cancer are ineffective and, in a few cases, dangerous. (Vitler, 1980)

Vitamin E has been touted for the prevention and treatment of heart disease, muscular weakness, cancer, ulcers, skin disorders, burns, and shortness of breath. Some have promoted its value for prolonging life, increasing vitality, and improving sexual performance. Here again, initially optimistic reports have been followed by studies that have failed to demonstrate any value of large doses of vitamin E in these conditions.

For instance, early work with laboratory animals showed that vitamin E was necessary for preventing sterility in male rats and for maintaining normal pregnancy in female rats who were denied the vitamin in their diet. It was therefore thought that vitamin E might have a role in the treatment of human infertility, spontaneous abortion or impotence. However, after more than 35 years of research, vitamin E has never been shown to be useful for any of these purposes. In other words, the deficiency produced by denying vitamin E to rats does not imply any value to additional vitamin E for humans who already have an adequate intake. This also applies to the treatment and prevention of heart disease. (Herbert, 1980)

Vitamin E deficiency is rare. The vitamin is present in many foods normally found in the diet: cereals, meat, fish, poultry, milk, eggs, legumes, fruits and nuts. In some uncommon illnesses—infant prematurity, intestinal malabsorption, retrolental fibroplasia, encephalopathies and chemical toxicity—vitamin E supplementation may be beneficial. Fortunately, taking supplements of vitamin E does not appear to pose a significant health risk. It is, however, largely a waste of money that could be better spent on wholesome food.

Vitamin A is found in carotenoids, which are converted to the active vitamin in the intestine. It is essential for the growth and maintenance of normal epithelial tissue (the tissue that covers the skin surface and lines the body cavities), and its deficiency produces night-blindness and drying, thickening and destruction of the conjunctiva (the mucous membrane that lines the eyeball and inside of the eyelids). Vitamin A deficiency may also produce abnormalities in the intestinal tract, lungs and urinary system. However, because vitamin A is found in meat, fish, oils, eggs, butter, cream and green leafy and yellow vegetables, its deficiency is extremely unlikely to occur with any diet that contains an adequate supply of calories.

Intoxication with vitamin A—which, like vitamin E, is fat-soluble—is a major potential health hazard. In doses of 150,000 units per day (30 times the recommended amount)—which are sometimes taken by vitamin enthusiasts—vitamin A can produce blurred vision, blindness, anorexia, and liver and bone damage.

Pregnant women who ingest large supplements of vitamin A may induce malformations (hydrochephalus, encephalocele) in their fetuses' nervous systems while children taking supplementary vitamin A in large doses may develop a neurological disease called pseudomotor cerebri, in which the symptoms mimic those of a brain tumor. And although vitamin A has been used to prevent experimentally induced tumors in laboratory animals, it has not been shown to prevent cancer in humans.

In recent years, some prevalent myths have apparently promoted vitamin supplementation. For example, there is no indication that women taking birth control pills need or will benefit from supplemental folic acid or vitamin B_6. Nor is there any evidence that smokers should take supplemental vitamin C or that this vitamin will prevent lung cancer. Some research indicates that smokers do occasionally have lowered levels of vitamin C, but these same studies also show that these levels are within the normal range.

The Cost of Vitamin Supplements

Vitamin supplements, whether prescribed by a proponent of megadose therapy, or suggested by a health-food-store proprietor, can be extremely expensive. For instance, a 48-year-old man with hypertension and a poor record of compliance with conventional medications was advised by a health-food-store operator to switch to "natural" treatment. He was sold 18 different types of tablets, with a total daily intake of 61 pills. The annual cost of these supplements and vitamins, which included such diverse substances as calcium pangamate, manganese, multi-vitamins, casein hydrolysate and desiccated liver extract, came to more than $1,000. This was at least 5 times what conventional antihypertensive therapy would have cost. Moreover, not a single one of these substances has been shown to be effective treatment for hypertension.

This example is extreme only in that the individual in this case was taking nutritional supplements for a medical problem not likely to respond to this approach. The fact that the cost was very high is not surprising. Nutritional supplements sold in health-food stores are often vended at extremely inflated prices. One of the great deceptions practiced in the alternative drug industry is the selling of products that are labeled as "natural" for many times what they are actually worth. Dollar for dollar, consumers would obtain better nutritional value by investing these resources in wholesome food. Those who insist on adding vitamins to their diet should purchase them at a reduced cost in supermarkets or other establishments not touted as "health food" stores.

Finally, the products sold as "stress vitamins" do not in any way reduce or prevent stress. They are also usually more expensive in this form, and are therefore an additional waste of money. All vitamin products must meet the same FDA standards of potency and purity.

Vitamins in Psychiatric Illness

During the mid-1950's psychiatry began to be interested in the potential role of vitamins in treating various mental disorders including schizophrenia and depression, and minimal brain dysfunction (MBD) and hyperkinetic behavior in children. In 1954 Drs. Abraham Hoffer and Humphrey Osmond published, in the *Journal of Mental Sciences,* the results of a year's research into the use of vitamin B_3 (also known as nicotinic acid, nicotinamide, and niacin) in the treatment of schizophrenia. They reported an improvement in the condition of the patients who were treated with the vitamin, and argued that the treatment had favorably altered biochemical reactions within the brain that were responsible for the hallucinations and other disordered thought processes characteristic of the disease. Unfortunately, their research was in many respects—including placebo factors—not well controlled.

Follow-up studies using niacin in schizophrenia failed to show any usefulness of the vitamin for this disease. Yet despite this, a branch of therapy known as "orthomolecular psychiatry" was born. In 1968 public and professional interest in orthomolecular methods was further enhanced by Dr. Linus Pauling in an article published in *Science* (Pauling,

1968). In this report he hypothesized that even in the face of a normal diet, individual differences in genetic make-up and food metabolism could create undetected imbalances and deficiencies in the body's chemistry. Therefore, wrote Pauling, some patients needed an approach which included ". . . the treatment of mental disease by the provision of the optimum molecular environment for the mind, especially the optimum concentration of substances normally present in the human body."

Numerous studies, attempting to prove this theory, have consistently failed to show that vitamin administration is useful in treating psychiatric illness. The American Psychiatric Association's Task Force on Vitamin Therapy in Psychiatry drew the following conclusion:

> In our view the results and claims of the advocates of megavitamin therapy have not been confirmed by several groups of psychiatrists and psychologists experienced in psychopharmacological research. The negative results have been obtained with adequately sized populations, employing careful observations by physicians, psychologists, and nurses and employing standards, reliable psychological and behavioral rating scales and appropriate statistics. (Task Force Report, 1973).

The enthusiastic early reports of the orthomolecular psychiatrists were overly optimistic, and idealistically underestimated the chemical complexity of psychiatric illness.

Pangamic Acid and Laetrile

Probably the most devious and unconscionable misrepresentation of vitamin therapy has been in the promotion of laetrile (amygdalin, or vitamin B_{17}—although it is not even remotely a vitamin) and pangamate (pangamic acid or vitamin B_{15}). As noted earlier, these substances are not vitamins, nor have they ever been shown to have any positive role in human nutrition or in the treatment or prevention of any illness. Both are potentially toxic. Laetrile contains cyanide (6% by weight), which is a deadly poison, while pangamate is a heterogeneous substance that often contains one or more potential poisons. Actually—because it is a variable mixture of chemical substances—there is no such thing as pangamate, and in some states it has been seized by law enforcement officials. The Canadians have prohibited its sale.

In 1943 Ernest Krebs Sr. and Ernest Krebs Jr., both laetrile proponents, applied for patent rights to pangamic acid. They claimed that it would "detoxify toxic products formed in the human system" and would be useful in providing immunity and treating a variety of disorders including asthma, skin diseases, respiratory tract illnesses, painful nerve and joint disease, arthritis, eczema and neuritis. When the Krebses applied for this patent there was not one shred of controlled experimental evidence that supported these claims. Almost 40 years later, this proof is still lacking. (Herbert, July, 1979)

On the other hand, one of the potential constituents of pangamate—diisopropylamine—can produce lowered blood pressure (hypotension) and lowered body temperature (hypothermia), cyanosis, and respiratory failure. Dichloroacetate, also found in some pangamate preparations, is a potential mutagen, and is therefore capable of producing both birth defects and cancer.

The proponents of pangamate appear to be shady, unreliable and unscrupulous. Ernest Krebs Jr. has attempted to pass himself off as a doctor, yet has no medical degree. His "honorary" doctorate in science comes from American Christian College in Tulsa, Oklahoma, which has no science department and is not empowered by the state of Oklahoma to grant the degree. Andrew McNaughton, head of the McNaughton Foundation, which has promoted both pangamate and laetrile, has been convicted of stock fraud. Dr. Victor Herbert commented on both men in the *American Journal of Clinical Nutrition:*

> Andrew McNaughton appears to be a laetrile factory owner with two criminal convictions, and Krebs appears to be a medical school flunkout with at least one criminal conviction. They appear to interact closely in promoting B_{15} and B_{17}. (Herbert, May, 1979)

The laetrile story is even more disquieting. Despite the fact that it has never been demonstrated in scientific studies to have any therapeutic or nutritional value, it has been sold worldwide as both a vitamin (B_{17}) and a cure for cancer, and has become a billion-dollar-plus yearly business. And it has been associated with at least 16 deaths.

Laetrile proponents point out that normal cells of the body contain an enzyme, rhodanase, which is capable of converting the cyanide in laetrile to thiocyanate. Since this enzyme is not present in cancer cells, they argue that it is an ideal form of treatment. However, rhodanase does not completely detoxify the cyanide in laetrile, and the thiocyanate (a sulfur-containing cyanide substance) is also toxic. Furthermore, there is no evidence that amygdalin kills tumor cells in preference to normal cells.

Ernest Krebs Sr. appears to have begun using laetrile in cancer treatment in the United States as early as the late

1920's. This was not its first use for this purpose (it had been used for 40 years before), but it was highly significant because both Krebs Sr. and Krebs Jr. were to be influential in its later promotion. In 1951 Ernest Krebs Jr. developed a purified form of laetrile that could be injected directly into the blood stream, and a few years later promoted an oral form that could be more readily dispensed to patients.

From the beginning, the use of laetrile as a cancer treatment has been shrouded in political debate. On April 20, 1970, the FDA granted the McNaughton Foundation permission to investigate laetrile in the treatment of cancer. Under pressure, the FDA rescinded the permission 1 week later. In their denial of the Investigative New Drug (IND) application for laetrile (which is required for all prospective new drugs) the FDA cited a number of deficiencies that the McNaughton Foundation actually tried to respond to. Despite this, the FDA formally rejected the application on May 12, 1970. They stated that laetrile had never been shown to be safe or efficacious, and that there was some question about the medical practitioners who would be conducting the research. They further argued that the IND application failed to delineate exactly how the drug worked. Laetrile proponents replied that aspirin, penicillin, and tranquilizers had all been approved for clinical investigation without full elaboration of their mechanism of action. The dispute appeared to be a political one between alternative medicine and the establishment.

The political furor over laetrile continues today, amidst considerable public interest over its use as a cancer treatment. Thousands of people with serious cancers flee to clinics in Mexico, Germany and the Caribbean for treatment. But while some states have legalized laetrile, the allopathic medical profession continues to be unalterably opposed to its use. Unfortunately, patients who seek laetrile treatment abroad do so in completely unregulated medical settings. In Mexico, for instance, some clinics apparently dispense steroids, nonsteroidal antiinflammatory agents and tranquilizers in conjunction with the therapy; and there have been a number of hospital admissions for poisoning associated with the therapy.

Under considerable public pressure the National Cancer Institute authorized four centers, The Mayo Clinic in Rochester, Minnesota, the University of California at Los Angeles, the University of Arizona Health Sciences Center in Tucson, Arizona and the Memorial Sloan-Kettering Cancer Center in New York, to conduct a clinical trial of laetrile in cancer patients. The results of the study were first publicized at the annual meeting of the American Cancer Society in Washington, D.C., in May, 1981.

The clinical trial included 178 patients with advanced cancer who had no other available therapy left open to them (using laetrile in lieu of a known therapy with potential effectiveness could not be justified on ethical grounds). One-third of the patients had already received chemotherapy but had failed to respond. They were given laetrile intravenously for 21 days, followed by oral doses. The researchers claimed that they were using the typical therapy regimen of the Mexican laetrile clinics. The patients were also given a diet of fresh fruits and vegetables and whole grains, as well as added vitamins and minerals. As might be expected, there was a placebo effect; 19% of the patients reported feeling better at some time in the study, but by 10 weeks only 5% still reported feeling improved.

The results of the study failed to show any benefit

from the laetrile therapy for any of the patients. Their tumors did not regress, their symptoms failed to improve and their survival was not extended. By 3 months' time, 90% of the patients showed evidence of progression of their cancer. By 8 months only 20% of the patients were left alive. The research team resoundingly pronounced laetrile a failure in treating cancer. Yet despite the results of this study, laetrile is unlikely to disappear from the cancer debate in the near future.

William D. Kelley, a graduate of the dental school at Baylor University in Texas, has promoted another form of "nutritional therapy" for cancer. The "Kelley diet" uses coffee enemas, pancreatic enzyme supplements (which can dissolve normal human tissue), hydrochloric acid tablets, comfrey-pepsin, raw juices and vegetables and amygdalin. Dr. Kelley's claims for both the prevention and treatment of cancer through dietary therapy have been grandiose, anecdotal and unproven. In an interview for *The Healthview Newsletter,* a publication that promotes unconventional nutritional therapy, he said:

> If a person has about three months to live, a well-designed nutritional program can give him or her slightly better than a 50-50 chance of survival. If the person has six months to go, recovery should be almost routine. With the research on nutrition that's now available, almost all early cancer patients—maybe 98 out of 100—can be saved. (*Healthview Newsletter,* 1977)

Kelley is not a trained cancer specialist. As a dentist, one can only guess where his background for cancer treatment (or any kind of medical care not related to dentistry) comes from. His evidence has never been independently examined by the scientific community, nor have his "cures" ever been documented in controlled clinical studies. Besides the deaths noted from coffee enemas, pancreatic enzyme supplements are potentially dangerous because they can damage normal tissue, and hydrochloric acid tablets can produce or aggravate ulcers.

Homeopathy

During the lifetime of its founder, Dr. Samuel Hahnemann, homeopathy spread throughout the world. His writings were translated into French, Latin, German, English, Italian, Russian and Hungarian. By 1851 there were 109 text books on homeopathy in English, homeopathic medical journals, and approximately 3,000 practitioners. Homeopathic hospitals existed in the United States, Spain, Poland, Russia, Turkey, Germany, Austria and Italy.

Homeopathy came to America in the mid-1820's, when Constantine Herring, a Philadelphia physician (1800–1850) credited with being the father of American homeopathy, proposed that a set pattern of symptoms indicated both illness and cure. This became known as Herring's Law. Significantly, the first national medical society in America was the American Institute of Homeopathy, founded in 1844.

From the beginning, homeopathy upheld the motto "Cure with safety," and like the Thomsonian herbalists, saw itself as a reaction to the "heroic" allopathic methods of blistering, leeching and bleeding. Homeopathic treatment was also less expensive than allopathic care. For instance, the hospital for orphan girls in Nice, France, reported that prior to 1838 the average annual cost of medicine was 416 francs.

With the introduction of homeopathy in 1839 this cost was reduced to 80 francs annually. By 1840 the hospital claimed to have spent only 10 francs on medicine.

However, in the twentieth century, bitter opposition from allopathic medicine forced the closure of schools for homeopathic training. This ultimately produced a rapid decline in the popularity of homeopathy. Even Hahnemann Medical College in Philadelphia, named after the founder of homeopathy, stopped teaching courses in its science. Although most practicing homeopaths today are trained allopathic physicians, there are no conventional medical schools that teach the method. In Britain, where the government provides funds for postgraduate medical training, these monies cannot be used for homeopathic education.

Nevertheless, homeopathy survived, and in recent years has seen an upsurge in interest, presumably catalyzed by the growth of the entire alternative healing industry. In 1978 the Federal Republic of Germany established a separate register for homeopathic remedies, thereby giving homeopathy independent legal status. In 1970 Sri Lanka (Ceylon) recognized homeopathic practice. India has a few homeopathic training institutions, and Pakistan has given recognition to the practice.

However, homeopathy is today a purely descriptive, or empirical discipline. One reason for this may be that homeopathy, beginning with Hahnemann himself and continuing with his followers, tested its thousands of plant and mineral substances on *normal* human subjects. They apparently never saw the need to devise clinical trials to test for effectiveness or placebo response. The *Journal of the American Institute of Homeopathy,* for example, carries one anecdotal report after another, but no studies that would currently pass as scientific papers. Surprisingly this empirical tradition continues despite the fact that today's homeopaths are physicians, trained in the allopathic mode of clinical investigation.

In an article that appeared in the *Journal of the American Institute of Homeopathy* in 1980, for instance, Dr. Lucy Clark described the treatment of grief with 5 homeopathic remedies. She reported the use of these substances based on the *symptoms* for which they should be employed. Thus, grief accompanied by feelings of suicide, a dislike for sympathy from others, and associated with symptoms of a cold and aggravated during the daytime should be treated with *Aurum* (gold). On the other hand, grief in the person who prefers to cry in solitude, dislikes sympathy from others, feels better in the open air and dislikes salt should be treated with *Natrum Mur* (a plant substance). A client who cries readily, craves sympathy, has no thirst, and who feels worse with heat should, however, be treated with *Pulsatilla* (a plant substance). There is no way of applying current scientific methods of evaluation to this kind of presentation. The patients' sex, age, severity of symptoms are not described. There is no mention of how data were collected, or of standard control groups. We do not know what, if any, hypothesis is being tested. In short, this bears no relationship to modern forms of scientific investigation.

The Theory of Homeopathy

Herring's Law—which taught that the symptoms of illness progressed in severity from outward to inward, and from below the waist to above the waist—amplified Hahnemann's view that the symptoms of an illness were the body's manifestation of an internal disorder of harmony in the vital force *(elan vital),* and that symptoms were actually a positive demonstration of the body's effort to heal itself of this internal disorder. According to Herring's Law, the more serious the illness the deeper it went into the body. The most serious illness was psychological illness, which had penetrated deep into the brain and up to the top of the body.

Herring's Law holds that curing illness involves reversing this process, and that the signs of cure progress from within outward. Thus, a skin eruption might be the final manifestation of an illness. Furthermore, homeopaths believe that the symptoms of illness are an integral part of the healing process (restoration of order in the vital force); they oppose any drugs or treatments which suppress symptoms. This includes steroids and other antiinflammatory medications. Instead, homeopathic remedies are designed to bring out symptoms, and people undergoing homeopathic treatment often experience a "healing crisis" at the beginning of therapy in which their symptoms appear to worsen.

Homeopaths point to the similarity between remedies and immunization in allopathy. Diphtheria and polio immunizations, for instance, are injections of detoxified substances that stimulate the body's immunological system and prevent disease. However, this comparison is purely conjectural in its relationship to homeopathic remedies, which are given after the person is already ill. Further, it is difficult to see the resemblance between a remedy that may be used in a variety of illnesses to the inactivated polio virus—for example—which stimulates immunity to polio, and only polio.

Perplexing also is that homeopathy has an entirely different set of diagnostic categories from allopathy. For instance, one does not have asthma, but an array of highly individualized symptoms that demonstrate disorder in the *elan vital.* Because of this, two people with asthma may receive entirely different remedies. One person may receive a remedy that—as noted earlier—is for symptoms that are aggravated by cold, accompanied by thirst and aggravated tension, while another asthmatic will receive a remedy based on fatigue in the morning, a ready tendency to sweat, and the avoidance of food. This is, again, a throwback to an earlier form of medicine, when healers knew little about the *underlying* cause of disease and treated only its symptoms.

Homeopathy and the Placebo Effect

Possibly the most puzzling of all aspects of homeopathy is its belief that the *smaller* the dose of a remedy the more potent it is. In fact, the most potent remedies have been so diluted that they can no longer be found by any conventional assay technique in the liquid vehicle in which they are administered. Arndt's Law, one of the basic tenets of homeopathy, states that a small amount of a remedy stimulates a healing reaction, a moderate amount of a remedy modifies the reaction (not particularly desirable), and a large amount suppresses the reaction (definitely undesirable). Homeopathic remedies of the 30th dilution—considered extremely *potent*—contain neither "ions nor electrons" of the remedy "left in the solution." (Stephenson, 1960)

In other words, in taking the most potent homeopathic remedies, one is taking in only water or some other liquid vehicle. Homeopaths argue that the remedy has altered the "energy" of the vehicle in some important way that promotes a healing reaction. However, to conventional healers, this confirms that homeopathy is, in effect, a large-scale placebo exercise. Homeopathic remedies are often sold as microdilutions impregnant upon sugar pills. If this were done in allopathic practice it would be considered placebo administration. Again, it is curious that physicians with an allopathic background make up the majority of homeopathic practitioners in Western nations.

Two attempts to study the effectiveness of homeopathy in controlled tests have failed to show any significant effectiveness in the approach. The first trial, performed in Britain, compared homeopathic and allopathic treatments of rheumatoid arthritis. The patients were divided into two treatment groups plus a placebo group that was used as a control. One treatment group received high-dose aspirin therapy while the other received a variety of homeopathic remedies. At the end of 1 year, the major finding was that the dropout rate in the aspirin group was high and that the homeopathy group was more able to tolerate its therapy. However, the study was not done in a double-blind fashion (to eliminate healer bias), and both groups of patients were free to take nonaspirin antiinflammatory agents. The experimental design was criticized widely for its methodological flaws, and a second trial was attempted.

In this second study, patients were again assigned to aspirin (plus nonaspirin antiinflammatory agents) or a homeopathic remedy (plus nonaspirin antiinflammatory agents), but this time administration of the treatments was done in a double-blind manner. Unfortunately, the study was conducted only over a 3-month period, which is generally considered too short for a chronic disease like rheumatoid arthritis (which typically has periods of exacerbation and remission), and involved only 23 patients in each group.

The authors found a slight improvement in the homeopathically treated group, but there was no way of knowing what the effect of the nonaspirin antiinflammatory agents was. It is surprising that the study allowed the use of symptom-suppressing antiinflammatory drugs, since homeopaths are traditionally opposed to these medications. Moreover, one of the basic principles of homeopathy is to try to employ only one remedy at a time, so that the use of several drugs in concert in the study is somewhat perplexing. While both studies indicate the type of study needed to prove the effectiveness of homeopathy, neither particularly supports it as an important form of therapy.

Homeopathy does provide a good model for holistic care. Its practitioners pride themselves in taking extremely detailed client histories, and thereby spend a considerable amount of time with their clients. They are particularly interested in emotional and spiritual factors, rarely relying on physical examination and laboratory tests to make a diagnosis. Further, by claiming that the client's treatment is unique, and based solely on the client's individual symptoms, homeopathy reinforces the value of healer-client interaction. And since homeopaths claim to attempt to restore the vital force or energy within the client, they build upon spiritual concepts held by a significant portion of the public that is already critical of "scientific" allopathy.

In conclusion, the evaluation of the alternative drug therapies differs from that of the nondrug therapies because they involve taking a drug, which is a potentially dangerous affair. Any form of medicinal therapy (including the use of a placebo) poses the question of risk versus reward, and when the potential for reward has not been demonstrated in controlled experiments (and few if any of the alternative drug therapies have been adequately tested in this way), the risk—no matter how small—is unacceptable. Moreover, there is little regulatory control over the administration and proliferation of these therapies. Given this laissez-faire climate, the consumer would do well to heed the ancient advice of *Caveat emptor!*

chapter 7

Choosing an Alternative Healer

Choosing a healer, either conventional or unconventional, may be the most difficult of all consumer choices. In contrast to obtaining other services, health-care decisions are usually made in troubled times, when there is pain, illness or great emotional stress. Because of this, decisions are often made in a desperate, hasty or impractical fashion. Therefore, even the most cautious consumer may make poor decisions.

But choosing an alternative healer is even more difficult than choosing a conventional one. There are few rules with which to guide the consumer. One can try to make a match on the basis of fees, the availability of appointment time, proximity of geographical location, and the referral of trusted friends, but these factors do not guarantee the *quality* of care.

It is distressing that people often choose a healer on the basis of word-of-mouth recommendation from friends, or from articles and advertisements in the popular press. These may be extremely unreliable. Friends often judge healers on the basis of such placebo-related factors as warmth, empathy, the appearance of the office and the courtesy of the ancillary staff. Articles in the popular press may be written by journalists more interested in finding a sensational story than accurately depicting the value of a new approach. Advertisements are virtually without any guarantee of honesty or accuracy. Periodicals take advertisements on the basis of the advertiser's ability to pay, not because of the proven value of a product or treatment.

The uncertainty of choosing has been further aggravated by the allopathic medical community's refusal to associate with alternative healers. Since the early 1800's, conventional practitioners have taken the view that association with alternative medical models tarnishes their practice. The continued anti-alternative message of the last 150 years has had the effect of diminishing the potential value of valid criticism of the alternative therapies by the allopathic medical establishment. It is easy for unconventional healers to claim that the system is a united front conspiring to restrain their competitive trade. As a result two opposing healing camps have unfortunately emerged, and the average consumer is caught between them.

How does one choose a healer? It is always prudent to begin with a complete investigation of your problem with a comprehensive medical interview, physical examination and laboratory tests performed by a licensed medical professional. In most cases, it is also sensible to have a trial with a standard form of medical therapy—unless, of course, the treatment plan is unacceptable for personal reasons.

Unconventional healers are not adequately trained in the diagnosis of serious illness. Because of this, they may miss potentially serious yet treatable diseases. And once such diagnoses are missed, early treatment of the disease may be delayed until therapy is no longer effective. Once you have a good idea of what your problem is, you can make better choices about how you want to deal with it.

Choosing a Healing Method

Before committing yourself to a specific approach, research what is known about its therapeutic effectiveness. The library of a medical college can be a valuable resource of articles that include valid clinical studies. A good medical librarian can help you find materials, and your conventional medical provider can aid you in understanding their content.

Whenever possible it is best to use an alternative approach that has already demonstrated some effectiveness. Hypertension, for example, has been shown to be amenable to biofeedback, meditation and relaxation techniques. While the exact amount of blood-pressure lowering cannot usually be predicted, and is known to depend on many individual factors, it is not altogether unfounded to try one of these methods. On the other hand, herbal remedies, chiropractic and acupuncture have not demonstrated usefulness in treating hypertension. Be aware that if you choose an unproven approach, you are likely to be operating largely on your own faith and the faith of the healer.

Pick a method that provides you with skills that you

can use on your own. One of the basic philosophical tenets of holism is that clients should maintain control over their own bodies. Thus, a preferable alternative therapy is one that keeps you in control, and gives you tools with which you can promote your own individual growth. The nondrug therapies such as relaxation and meditation fall into this category, as do exercise and nutritional programs that you can learn and use in your daily living. On the other hand, megavitamin therapy, homeopathy and chiropractic do not do this. The control remains in the hands of the therapist, and you remain dependent upon the therapist's services.

Choose a therapy that allows you to mix conventional and alternative methods. If you have hypertension, for instance, you can employ biofeedback or progressive relaxation in conjunction with your antihypertension medications. Eventually you may be able to lower your blood pressure enough to reduce your daily medication requirement, or even possibly eliminate it. But while you are learning the alternative method, you can still have the safety of continuing your medications. Be wary of any approach that says you must discontinue medicines that have been prescribed for a potentially serious medical disorder.

Consumers should also avoid cultism; this means any approach that says there is only *one* way to solve a problem. Many people do best with a variety of techniques ranging from nutritional approaches to massage and relaxation. In fact, the pluralism of the alternative model is one of its strong points. It allows an individual to seek out a number of choices and find the one or ones that are best for the individual's specific needs.

Healers who adopt the notion that their way must exclude all others may be dangerous. Dr. Richard Ingrasci of Interface, a holistic educational association in the Boston area, states that:

> There is a macrobiotic cult in Boston [which believes] that the answer to the world's problems is [in] macrobiotics. Sometimes people who go to holistic health [practitioners] are desperate, and some cancer patients go to the macrobiotic community and are told that you can cure cancer with brown rice and a macrobiotic diet. Some of these people get better and these are the ones that the cult members write up. But, as a health practitioner in the Boston area, I can tell you that a lot of them don't get better. Some get worse and die.
>
> What happens is that the community irresponsibly blames the victim. If you don't get better it is because you are not pure enough. You may not be eating the right food, or chewing it fifty times as you are supposed to. It's a Catch 22. They take no responsibility for failure. You can always have a terrific track record if you only pay attention to the successes and ignore the failures.

In short, avoid zealots and therapies that force you to exclude potentially beneficial methods. Keep in mind that it is extremely rare for only one approach to be helpful.

Another useful guideline is to be suspicious of therapies that require you to sign up and pay in advance for a prescribed number of treatments. This approach locks you into a form of therapy. In some cases you may progress more rapidly than expected and not need the additional sessions. But, since you have paid for them, the healer is likely to ask you to complete the full course, so the healer can keep the full payment. On the other hand, if you are not progressing, you may nevertheless continue for the full treatment plan because you have already paid for the sessions. This may encourage you to stay with an unproductive therapy and delay your seeking other, potentially beneficial modes of treatment.

Finally, and most important, is to evaluate the potential *harm* of a method of treatment before agreeing to participate in it. Since all medicine is a question of risk versus reward, one should always try to minimize risk. Any form of treatment that involves taking untested, nonstandardized drugs or botanicals represents a potential risk that should be carefully considered. Coffee enemas and purgatives that disturb the normal internal balance of salts and water (fluids and electrolytes) fall into this category. So do mechanical devices, especially those that pass an electrical current through the body. Moreover, any very unconventional form of dietary therapy may involve the ingestion of potentially poisonous substances.

Choosing an Alternative Healer

A medical practitioner should satisfy the client's needs for caring and communication, as well as providing healing expertise. Studies of chiropractors, naturopaths and other unconventional healers repeatedly point to their clients' appreciation of their warmth and understanding. However, this is too often the major quality upon which a choice is made, and expertise is not adequately evaluated.

Consumers should be aware that a typical characteristic of hucksters and charlatans is an overly ingratiating and sensitive interpersonal approach. While it is valid to criticize the cold manner that is too often stereotypical of the allopathic practitioner, it is equally important to realize that excessive warmth and sensitivity are signs of a sales technique. Healers who exhibit these characteristics may be cultivating placebo factors, but they are also covering up their lack of technical expertise. Try to find a person who understands you and your problem, and who also has the technical competence to help you. Healing is an art, but it is also a skill that is learned through extensive training and practice.

You can begin by evaluating the practitioner's credentials and background. Since most alternative healing does not require state licensure, there may be a large variability in the training and expertise of healers. Some may be trained physicians who have taken on unconventional forms of practice, while others may have no formal medical background whatsoever. Some may be graduates of chiropractic programs or acupuncture schools, which provide a limited level of medical training. Be especially wary of people who have little training and claim to have a "lay" background. Dr. Jerome Schofferman of the Alternative Therapies Unit of San Francisco General Hospital advises:

> You should always ask the person that you are going to see what their background is. That means their credentials and experience. Find out if they have taken more than a two week workshop and now call themselves a practitioner. Find out what level of knowledge they have, who they have studied with, and how many patients they have worked with who have a problem similar to yours.

Be critical of the answers you get. People who claim to have seen "many, many cases just like yours" may not be telling the truth. Unfortunately, it is easy to make grandiose claims when you do not have to back them up with hard facts. Inquire as to whether they have published any of their evidence, or whether they can provide references who will support their claims. Ask others, including conventional professionals, to give their view of both the published articles and references. You can get a more balanced view by asking a few sources their opinion of the healer and the healing method.

Try to avoid people who say things like "Only I can help you," or "You have come to the best place." They are likely to be trying to sell you on their services by making unsubstantiated claims. With regard to this, Dr. Schofferman says:

> Ask the practitioner about how effective the therapy is, and be wary of anybody who says that it works for most everybody. Look for people who are honest and [say they] have an approach that . . . works for some people. They should have the attitude that "we will give it a try." Realize that people who make big promises rarely can keep them. Also be wary of people who sell chemicals and vitamins, even if they claim they are selling them at no mark-up.

Be critical of people who cannot explain what they are doing in a clear, concise and concrete fashion. Maintain a healthy skepticism of approaches that are vague and unscientific, such as those characterized by statements like "I am balancing your body energy" (often claimed by practitioners of Oriental medicine), or "I am returning you to alignment" (proposed by chiropractors). These concepts have never been demonstrated in any formal, scientific manner. They are being proposed as articles of faith. Practitioners should explain their methods in terms you can understand. The practitioner who says "It is hard to explain because it is very complicated," may really be indicating that he or she has only a vague concept of what he or she is doing.

Find someone who has expertise and experience in

both allopathic and alternative camps. This means physicians, trained psychologists, and in some cases mid-level practitioners (like physician assistants and nurse practitioners) who have received *additional* training in their alternative field of interest. Also try to find a group practice, where professionals blend a number of conventional and alternative skills.

Another safeguard is to choose a healer who is associated with a hospital or licensed clinic. That association may help in providing accountability for the quality of the services that are delivered. The supervising institution can provide an appeal process for problems related to inadequate care or incompetent practice.

The Alternative Therapies Unit at San Francisco General Hospital is a good example of a responsible alternate health-care facility. The practitioners at the Unit are accountable because they must be responsible to the hospital, its medical staff and its board of directors. Complaints or questions concerning services can be addressed to the hospital's department of medicine or board of directors. The practitioners in the Unit can also draw on the resources of the other professionals in the hospital. The hospital affiliation further guarantees that the practitioners have a minimum level of training and that their credentials have been reviewed by other health professionals.

Solo practitioners, not associated with any institution, remain immune to review by independent observers. If they are physicians, complaints may be addressed to the state's board of medical examiners, but these boards are limited in their ability to pursue questions of quality of care. It is even more difficult to get accountability from nonphysician healers.

Lastly, be particularly suspicious of people who call

themselves "doctor" but do not have a valid medical degree. They may claim to be a doctor of naturopathic, chiropractic, or Oriental medicine, or to have a degree in psychology or one of the "pure" sciences (like chemistry or biology). None of these degrees is associated with the level of medical training usually expected of allopathic physicians. While practitioners who call themselves "doctor" may be competent in what they do, they may also be using the term "doctor" to fool the public. Some, like Ernest Krebs, Jr., may have obtained mail-order or other suspicious doctorate degrees. Diploma mills that provide these degrees do not give any training that will help in the practice of healing. These practitioners are misrepresenting themselves to promote their business and your faith in their methods.

If you are uncertain about the background of your practitioner, you can contact the department of consumer affairs, department of public health or medical licensing agency in your state. They should be able to check on the qualifications of the practitioner. They may also be able to help you with any grievances you have about the quality of the care you receive. But remember that the best protection is always a cautious, alert and knowledgeable consumer. If you have *any* uncertainty about the healer, find another practitioner.

Making a Healing Contract

Some of the uncertainty involved in choosing an alternative healer can be eliminated with a clear agreement that delineates he roles of both client and practitioner. Contracts are our standard means of establishing agreements between informed individuals, and they can be applied to the healing arts just as they are in business and marriage.

Jerry Green, an attorney in Marin County, California, has written extensively on the use of contracts in the healing arts. He is particularly interested in their applicability to new areas of health care. In Green's view, health-care contracts can help eliminate the misunderstandings that produce malpractice actions and consumer disappointment.

The basic elements of a healing contract should be agreed upon prior to initiating a course of therapy. The contract should specify the goals of the healer-client relationship and the basic responsibilities of both parties, and should define the length of time that the agreement will be in effect. The contract does not necessarily have to be written, but is based on the communicated goals and responsibilities set forth by both parties. In other words, according to Green, "Verbal statements, notes of conversations, correspondence, or the behavior of the parties all evidence a contract. The contract exists in the minds of the parties."

For example, take a hypothetical healing contract for the treatment of hypertension. In setting forth the goals, the client would spell out the level of blood pressure that he or she would want by the end of the treatment course. This could then become a common purpose for both the healer and the client. The practitioner would take on the job only if he or she felt that the goal was reasonable given the healer's expertise. The length of time would be clearly defined in months, and an agreement would be made about when the contract would be reviewed by both the healer and the client.

The contract would also clarify how the therapy

would be conducted. The healer would say whether or not the client would continue taking any pre-contract medications, and would specify the activities related to the treatment plan. For hypertension, these might include a program of diet, exercise, stress reduction and the therapeutic method to be used. In turn, the client would agree to engage in these activities as directed by the healer. The healer would agree to provide a set number of sessions, to charge a certain fee and to provide regular blood pressure recording. The two parties might also agree that the healer would be available for telephone consultation.

One interesting aspect of this agreement is its application to the basic principles of holistic health care. The typical informed consent agreement in allopathic practice is designed to protect a relatively passive client. It spells out the nature of the treatment and its possible dangers and side effects, and describes alternative forms of therapy. But it still assumes that it is the patient who is being treated *by* the practitioner. In the contract proposed by Green, there is a sense of mutual responsibility and participation.

The novelty of this contractural process demands that it be implemented slowly and cautiously. It is not designed to be a basis for malpractice claims or other legal actions against healers. It functions primarily to clarify goals and obligations in a new and largely unregulated area of health care.

You do not need to come up with a contract in your first meeting with a healer. It may take a few sessions before you understand clearly what both you and the healer can accomplish together. However, when you do reach an agreement, you can commit it to writing in a letter that you send the healer. In this letter, state simply and clearly what you understand the basic elements of your agreement to be: your common goal, mutual responsibilities and the time period of the agreement. Keep the letter as a record of your contractual agreement.

In your letter you may also request certain basic information about the healer. This might include a description of the healer's training and background, the philosophy of the healer's practice, and a description of the healer's methods. You may also want to be specific about the number of sessions that are likely to be needed, the length of each session, the cost of each visit and whether there is a minimum number of treatments that the healer feels are necessary.

For instance, if you are being treated for hypertension, your healer may say that the first session includes a detailed history, physical examination and some blood and urine tests. The healer may also specify that this visit will last from 1 to 1½ hours and cost 50 dollars, while subsequent visits may last approximately 30 minutes and cost 20 dollars. In these subsequent sessions the healer may state that he or she will teach you a basic relaxation program, along with providing information concerning diet, exercise and stress reduction. The "contract" might state that the relationship usually involves at least 5 training sessions, and that a periodic follow-up every 3 months to record blood pressure is important for the first year.

Both parties should set forth how the contract is to be terminated and the schedule of payments. You may also want to request information concerning possible dangers of the treatment and other alternative therapies that may be helpful.

In working out this kind of agreement you are increasing your likelihood of finding an honest practitioner, establishing reasonable goals, and maintaining yourself as an active participant in the healing relationship.

Evaluating Yourself as a Patient

Many alternative approaches are quite demanding of the client. It is unwise to undertake a biofeedback or meditation program, for example, if you are a person who is not willing to devote the necessary effort to the program. Remember that it is as important to be honest about your own limitations as it is to choose the right therapy and therapist.

Moreover, you should pick a method that you are comfortable with. Just because a friend or loved one encourages you to follow a healing practice does not mean that it is right for you. People often follow fads to their own detriment. Avoid choosing a method because it is *avant garde* or because it worked for a close friend. Your problem and your personality may be entirely different from that of another person. In other words, don't give up your independence. Being a coequal in the healing process means that you have to be honest about your limitations. There is nothing that says that your self-esteem is diminished if you are more likely to benefit from conventional therapy.

Screening Hucksters

As noted earlier, one sign of a huckster is an extremely warm and ingratiating manner. This is how the huckster catches consumers off their guard. Dr. Robert Derbyshire, a past member of the New Mexico Board of Medical Examiners, illustrated this point with the story of Fred Brant, a convicted felon who successfully passed himself off as a physician. In *The Health Robbers* Derbyshire described how Brant was able ingratiate himself to the people of a small, rural Texas community. Brant took on the alias of Dr. Reid L. Brown and:

> . . . moved to Texas where he obtained a license by endorsement and served for three years on the staff of the state hospital in Terrell, Texas. He then resigned and took his wife on a vacation trip. Stopping for a Coca-Cola in the small village of Groveton, Texas, he treated the injured leg of a child. He found that Groveton had long been without a doctor and its people were clamoring for medical care. "Dr. Brown" soon became established as the town physician and as a community leader. (Barrett and Knight, 1976)

Fred Brant's success was based largely on his warm and personable manner. His charade was discovered only by a chance computer check by a drug company. Interestingly, when Brant was challenged by the authorities, the townspeople rallied to his defense. He was described as a "prince of a medical man, license or no license," and a local grand jury refused to indict him. Dr. Derbyshire commented:

> What were the secrets of Freddie Brant's success as an impersonator? They were many, but the main ones were his readiness to refer any potentially complicated case to nearby towns, a personality which inspired confidence, and a willingness to take time to listen to his patients. (Barrett and Knight, 1976)

Be suspicious of practitioners whose main attributes are sincerity and understanding; they are the same qualities that one might be suspicious of in a used car salesman, but rarely come into question when we deal with health-care providers. This does not mean that our health-care practitioners should not be likeable people; however, they should not appear to be sincerely selling a product or themselves in their delivery of health-care services.

One should also be wary of providers who practice outside their formal training. Usually these practitioners tout nutritional methods for which they have little formal training. They promote hair analysis or computer analysis for nutritional imbalance, sell various types of nutritional supplements and claim to "balance body chemistry." The use of the term "doctor" by dentists and Ph.D.'s who offer these services is misleading. Dentists are trained in disorders of the teeth and gums. People with Ph.D.'s should work in their area of training.

Hair analysis has become popular as a method of detecting nutritional deficiency. However, it has never been demonstrated to be useful in this regard. The American Medical Association's Committee on Cutaneous Health and Cosmetics has said that hair analysis is not an accurate indicator of health or nutritional status. The technique is rendered inaccurate by a variety of common factors including natural hair color, hair dyes, chlorine in swimming pools, age and sex.

Consumers should also be skeptical of nonmedical healers, such as evangelistic faith healers who attempt to give medical advice. Eleven-year-old Wesley Parker, for instance, died because his parents believed a faith healer and took away his insulin. In some cases faith healers have produced "cures," which the scientific community usually attributes to placebo effects, but these have involved the use of prayer and the laying on of hands, and not the giving of medical advice. Don't trust anyone who suggests that you discontinue vital medicines or encourages you to reject surgery because God will heal you.

Avoid Gadgets

The history of medicine is littered with useless, sometimes harmful gadgetry that has been touted for weight loss, diagnosing illness, curing cancer and restoring vitality. Recently the "Relax-A-Cisor" was sold for weight reduction. This gadget passed small doses of electricity into the body to produce muscle spasm. It was not only useless for losing weight but was also potentially dangerous. The "E-meter" promoted by L. Ron Hubbard, originator of Scientology, and the "Diapulse" heat device are other unproven medical gadgets. Such gadgets play on the public's awareness of legitimate advances made in engineering, computers, telecommunication and medical science, but they invariably do little more than catalyze placebo effects.

Dr. Phillip R. Alper, Clinical Professor of Medicine at the University of California in San Francisco, provided a useful summary of tips to help distinguish unproven methods and hucksters from legitimate practitioners. In *The Health Robbers* he wrote:

> Quacks are the despair of "straight" physicians. They are often charming and project a feeling of greater-than-usual concern. A charismatic quack can produce a legion of adoring clients to testify on his behalf. But certain behavior should make you suspect that a doctor has *abandoned* medical science:
>
> —If a doctor claims to have a special machine or formula.

—If he makes blanket statements that surgery, x-rays or drugs do more harm than good.

—If he claims that other doctors are persecuting him, or are afraid of his competition.

—If he advertises or uses testimonials from patients to build his practice.

This does not mean that all nontraditional healers are hucksters, or that their methods are worthless. But with the explosion of new alternatives to conventional methods, consumers need to be more astute than before.

c—h—a—p—t—e—r—8

Regulation of Alternative Healing

The many alternative healing disciplines that have exploded over the last decade have challenged more than half a century of allopathic control of the healing arts. Battles have been fought in the courts, legislatures and regulatory agencies. Some actions have produced important victories, especially for chiropractic, acupuncture and the pro-laetrile lobby.

Five states now license independent practice (not supervised or associated with a physician) for acupuncturists. All 50 states now license the independent practice of chiropractors, and the federal government recently agreed to reimburse some chiropractic services under Medicaid and

Medicare. Some states have legalized laetrile. At least one case has been won by a lay homeopath, who continues to practice without physician supervision.

This trend marks a major reversal of legal policy. In effect, the legal system has acknowledged that there is a plurality of expertise in health care, and that nonallopathic disciplines have a valid place in the delivery of health-care services.

Defining the Practice of Medicine

Medicine, according to *Taber's Cyclopedic Medical Dictionary*, is "the art of preventing, caring for and assisting in the cure of disease and the care of the injured." Unfortunately, this broad definition, while accurate in the literary sense, has not been particularly helpful in the legal arena. In its breadth, it encompasses health-care practices that we do not normally associate with the practice of medicine by physicians. According to this definition, the mother who diagnoses a cold in her child and prescribes rest and fluids could be considered as practicing medicine without a license. Similarly the school nurse who teaches sex education could be considered as practicing medicine; or the friend who applies ice and an elastic bandage to an injured ankle might come under this broad definition. Even the preacher who cries out "Throw away your crutches and walk" could be considered to be practicing medicine.

Steve Samuels is a Boston area attorney who has become interested in the legal status of alternative healers. Like other observers, he has become concerned about the overly broad definition of medical practice inherited from an earlier era. Samuels says that:

> The practice of medicine has been defined by doctors and the medical establishment in the broadest of ways. Basically, if you ate part of my sandwich and then began to have stomach pains, and I asked you, "What did you eat?"; and if you reply, "A pastrami sandwich from the Hot Spot," and I say "Ah, I've seen that before. That pastrami is sometimes bad, and if you rest, do a little meditation and take Alka SeltzerT, you'll be fine," I will be practicing medicine.

For instance, the owner of a health-food store in Sacramento, California, was charged with practicing medicine without a license because she gave out nutritional advice. If this is practicing medicine, then even schools, in the nutritional advice they give, could be considered as practicing medicine. Similarly, the nutritional counseling that many holistic educators and healers provide could be considered as medical practice.

It has been in the interest of allopathic medicine to define the practice of medicine in such broad terms; the definition has encouraged a legal policy that can easily be used to exclude potentially competitive practitioners. It assumes that allopathic medicine, as taught in the medical schools in the United States and Europe, holds the ultimate authority on medical knowledge, and that legally, people with alternative expertise should be considered subservient to allopathy. However, some people in both the legal field and in alternative medicine are challenging this premise. According to Steve Samuels:

> The practice of medicine has been defined by state legislatures and court cases. In either case the people who are practicing medicine are primarily physicians. In case law the lawyers and judges generally rely on physicians' testimony

> to reach a judgement in the case. They abdicate their authority to the doctor who is supposed to know this area.
>
> This assumes that the only people who know anything about the body and health have been to an accredited medical school, which leaves out a lot of people. For instance, in [a recent] *New York Times* there was a story about the Dalai Lama's physician. It leaves him out. The Western doctors are somewhat shocked about how he makes a diagnosis, but it is the Western physicians who are doing something radically new. He has been doing his diagnosis based on a practice that is 4,000 years old, whereas we are doing it based on a practice that at most is a few hundred years old.

Many people have become skeptical of the notion that allopathy has a monopoly of healing expertise. In the California hearings on the question of independent licensure of acupuncturists, many speakers pointed out that acupuncture was a valid discipline that preceded Western allopathy by thousands of years. Herbalists and naturopaths cite that their methods also predate allopathic medicine. Furthermore, the legalization of laetrile in a number of states suggests that many people do not believe that the FDA and the National Cancer Institute have a monopoly of expertise in cancer treatment.

As yet, little has been resolved in reaching a more acceptable definition of the practice of medicine. Most states have medical practice statutes that define the practice of medicine extremely broadly. The California Medical Practice Act is an example of these laws. It states that:

> Any person who practices or attempts to practice, or who advertises or holds himself out as practicing, any system or mode of treating the sick or afflicted in this state, or who

> diagnoses, treats, or operates for any ailment, blemish, deformity, disease, disfigurement, disorder, injury, or mental or physical condition of any person, without having at the time of so doing a valid, unrevoked certificate . . . is guilty of a misdemeanor.

Some legal analysts would like to clarify this definition in light of the upsurge in interest in the nonallopathic healing arts. Attorney Jerry Green maintains that there is a basic difference between medicine as practiced by allopaths and healing as practiced by nontraditional practitioners. According to Green, allopathic medicine is the science of diagnosing and treating pathological conditions, while nonallopathic healing is based on an empirical tradition that does not deal directly with the pathological disorders usually treated by conventional medicine. In the process of rethinking the roles of both types of healers, Green had an opportunity to test his hypothesis in the Dana Ullman case that began in 1976.

In defending Ullman—the Oakland, California lay homeopath who was indicted under the California Medical Practice Act for practicing medicine without a license—Green argued that homeopathy had established itself more than 100 years earlier as a separate and valid empirical discipline. Citing the work of Harris Coulter, a medical historian, Green claimed that homeopathy regarded symptoms, pathology and the body's vital energy *(elan vital)* differently from allopathic medicine. He argued that because Ullman practiced a different form of healing, he should not have been considered as practicing medicine. In other words, while Ullman was engaging in a type of health practice, it was not the practice of medicine as defined by the medical practice statute. In an interview, Green commented:

> When I looked at the California statute that defines who can practice medicine, I realized that we could get greater clarity out of our medical relationships if we made agreements with doctors that defined their responsibility in terms of their science . . . [the Ullman case] was the first opportunity I had to test two hypotheses. The first, which we did not test because we did not go to trial, was that holistic practices are fundamentally different from the [allopathic] treatment of pathology. . . . And [the California Medical Practices Act] is conveniently written in terms that relate to pathology. It seems to paint a broad picture, but I interpret that to pertain to pathological conditions. If you did not interpret this narrowly—and it is a criminal statute—it would probably be unconstitutional. It would make any condition a person could imagine to be a medical one. And that is really not defining medicine at all.

Because Dana Ullman won his case without going to trial, no new definition of medical practice was proposed. We do not know whether the court accepted Green's argument that homeopathy had developed as a valid healing discipline separately and independently from allopathy, or whether there was another weakness to the state's case. Nor do we have further clarification of the boundaries of allopathic practice as distinct from the larger concept of health care.

For instance, is health teaching a form of medical practice as defined by current statute? Seemingly the indictment of a health-food-store owner for practicing medicine by giving out nutritional information appears to come under the law as interpreted in California. But if this is medical practice, then why is the nutritional advice offered by the school nurse or science teacher not medical practice? Similarly, is teaching biofeedback for the purpose of stress reduction practicing medicine? If not, then is it medical practice when it is taught for the treatment of a pathological condition like migraine headache or hypertension? Unfortunately, we do not yet have the answers to these questions.

Some of the new healers have tried to circumvent the law by claiming that their work does not treat illness. For instance, in a personal communication, Anna E. Hyder of the Rolf Institute wrote that: "Rolfing is not a medical treatment. . . . [W]e do not treat or diagnose pathological conditions. Rolfing is not a therapy or treatment of any kind and is not medical in nature."

Yet people go to Rolfers with many complaints that could be considered pathological, including musculoskeletal pain and emotional problems. Since "structural integration" as practiced by Rolfers is designed to release tension and shortening in the body's connective tissues, a strict reading of the California Medical Practice Act might consider this a treatment for "deformity, disease [and] disfigurement."

Similarly, a broad interpretation of medical practice could include the search for high-level well-being described by holists, who have sought a status independent of the medical practice statutes.

We need a new definition of medical care. Allopathy must be defined in terms of its own practices; and some compromise definition must be developed for nonallopathic practices. If we do not succeed in doing this we can look forward to many future battles, as healing disciplines look for a place in the delivery of health-care services.

Restraint of Trade

The compromise settlement in Dana Ullman's case did not permit him to practice medicine, nor did it help form a new and helpful definition of healing roles. And while it did allow him to continue his practice as a lay homeopath, it set specific conditions that were designed to prevent him from competing with physicians.

In the words of the legal settlement:

> Defendant [Mr. Ullman] has initiated a regular practice of contracting with clients in order to clarify the role of the *non-medical* [italics added] health practitioner and he encourages resort to licensed physicians for the diagnosis and treatment of pathology.

Ullman clearly comprehends that this does not permit him to practice medicine or compete with physicians in the delivery of medical services. He wrote that the settlement with the court "does *not* mean that all I have to do is say I'm not a doctor and then treat people . . . it does not mean that I can make a legal contract with my clients and then still diagnose and treat disease." (Ullman, 1978)

As has been stated throughout this book, the rise of the alternative healers has paralleled the public's suspicion of allopathic practice and the motivation of allopathic medicine for criticizing alternative healing methods. Consumers point out that medicine is big business and that its criticism of alternative health care is not always for public safety or altruistic reasons. Allopathic health care now costs the public about $200 billion annually, and physicians receive about 25% of this figure for services. In fact, doctors are the highest paid of all professionals, and the cost of health care continues to rise faster than the overall rate of inflation. Restrictive licensing laws have been the basis upon which allopathic practices have dominated the medical marketplace.

Critics point out that by restricting competition, allopathy keeps both its costs and fees high while having only a marginal effect in protecting the public. They claim that regulation is an economic and political issue, and not a matter of public safety. Samuels states that:

> The way that the practice of medicine has been defined is a political issue. It is only becoming a public [matter] now because of the economic issues. The reason that [this has] not come out before is that alternative healers are starting to take money away from traditional physicians.
>
> [Allopaths] will always say that they are concerned with . . . health and safety. . . . But why weren't they cracking down, for instance, on lay midwives before? Why is this an issue now? Clearly because it is taking money away from physicians, and they are . . . concerned about it.

Recently the Federal Trade Commission began to examine the question of restraint of trade in medical practice. In 1979 it found that the American Medical Association had violated the Federal Trade Commission Act in a number of ways. First, the AMA was clearly more like a trade association than a charitable or educational organization. The AMA operated to promote the economic gain of its members, and lobbied to obtain pro-physician legislation at the state and federal level. In addition, it conducted seminars designed to teach physicians to improve the efficiency and profitability of their practices. Moreover, it regularly provided legal advice on tax law and on how to set up model practice arrangements for economic purposes, and advised physicians on how to sell and dispose of existing medical practices.

The FTC also charged that the AMA had been involved in trying to establish fee scales that both controlled the marketplace and kept fees high. The Michigan State Medical Society, for instance, allegedly collected written proxies from physicians that allowed the Society to cancel participation in Blue Cross-Blue Shield and Medicaid if fee schedules were not set at acceptably high levels. In effect, medical societies worked to control prices for the benefit of allopathic practitioners.

The AMA was also criticized for its prohibition of physician advertising. The FTC felt that this was another example of how medical societies worked to keep fees high by restricting competition. While the AMA said that false advertising offered a potential public health danger, the FTC felt that the Association could instead promulgate and enforce ethical standards to protect the public. Thus, the AMA had options for preventing false or misleading claims other than by prohibiting physicians from making public their fees and services.

Finally, the FTC determined that the AMA should not prohibit physicians from forming partnerships with allied health practitioners. An example of this might be the partnership of a psychiatrist with a psychologist, or of an orthopedist with an acupuncturist. The AMA had discouraged this practice, claiming that nonphysicians might exert undue and detrimental influence on doctors.

Chiropractors have been the most active in seeking restraint of trade decisions against conventional medicine. In 1976 five chiropractors from different states filed suit in a Chicago court, charging that the AMA had worked to restrain their trade. Shortly afterward, similar actions were filed in New Jersey and Pennsylvania. Each action claimed that the AMA had attempted to monopolize medicine by creating an environment in which physicians had the sole opportunity to deliver health-care services.

The chiropractors' lawsuits stated that the AMA had adopted standards for practice that discouraged doctors from accepting chiropractic patients, or from performing X-ray services at the request of a chiropractor. They also pointed out that chiropractors had been excluded from practice in allopathic hospitals.

By 1978 the AMA apparently sensed a change in the political climate. Fearing that the chiropractors' lawsuits might end in a decision favorable to chiropractic, they withdrew their objection to physicians' providing diagnostic services for chiropractors, and passed new ethical codes which allowed physicians to take referrals from nonphysician practitioners. In doing so they reversed a tradition that was more than 150 years old.

The legal status of the nonphysician practitioners of alternative therapies remains unclear. In Texas, for instance, the Board of Medical Examiners passed regulations that restricted the practice of acupuncture to trained and licensed physicians. Recently, 46 residents of Harris County, Texas, filed suit, claiming that these regulations violated their right of access to medical services. At the time of the suit there were no licensed physicians practicing acupuncture in Texas, and no formal training programs for them to learn the art.

The litigants claimed that the action of the Board of Medical Examiners effectively denied them access to acupuncture services.

The Texas case is both a question of access to care and the right of allopathy to control nonallopathic services. The Board of Medical Examiners claimed that its regulations were designed to protect the public from misdiagnosis by nonphysicians, from injury due to the faulty placement of acupuncture needles and to assure that complications from therapy would be dealt with promptly and effectively. However, there is no evidence that nonphysician acupuncturists have been guilty of any of these faults or that physicians who provide acupuncture treatment are more qualified to do so than acupuncturists. While the case was not argued in terms of restraint of trade, it is an example of how restrictive regulation can control the marketplace. If physicians alone are permitted to provide alternative healing services, then the entire spectrum of healing arts will be restricted to practitioners trained first in allopathy.

The Role of Medical Supervision

In the last 15 years medicine has opened up to a small number of nonphysician medical providers. Physician assistants, nurse practitioners and midwives have been allowed by statute in most states to perform services normally associated with the practice of medicine. These mid-level practitioners, however, do not practice independently. In most situations they must be supervised by a physician. While this supervision does not necessarily mean that the doctor and practitioner see the same patients, or even work together in the same room, it does serve to keep control in the hands of physicians.

This might be an appropriate model for chiropractors, acupuncturists, holists, and other alternative healers. However, the alternative healers have resisted this form of legal restriction. Like Dana Ullman, many claim that their practices do not come under the scope of training and practice normally associated with allopathic medicine. They further reject any notion that their work should be reviewed by regulatory boards composed of physicians, or that certification or licensure should be based on standards established by allopaths.

In doing so the alternative healers argue that there is a plurality of expertise in health care. Medicine, they say, is only one way of looking at the human body and its problems; alternative practices represent an equally valid and different perspective on health. Jerry Green commented on this approach:

> Originally I thought holistic practice was going to be a new form of medicine; that it would indicate a new trend in medicine. But now as I see it, the bulk of this movement is outside the medical profession. The battle that will be fought over professional control will be between the physicians who want to control holistic practices and holistic practitioners, herbalists, midwives, nutritionists and others.

To date there have been few tests of this thesis. In *Maxwell* vs. *McCaffrey,* which was argued before the Virginia Supreme Court on March 2, 1979, the court refused to allow the testimony of an orthopedic surgeon in a malpractice suit against a chiropractor. In doing so the court acknowledged that the chiropractor and orthopedist practiced separate healing arts, and that the orthopedist did not hold expertise in chiropractic.

Nonallopathic healers favor the loosening of all licensing restrictions. Consumers would have the freedom to choose a licensed healer or a nonlicensed healer, and to make healing contracts that establish the parameters of care. Dana Ullman argues for a system that he calls "regulated freedom of choice," which, he says

> would allow people to consider going to certified health practitioners, to uncertified practitioners, or to themselves. It would be legal for uncertified practitioners to provide any service requested by their clients, except possibly for the use of potentially life threatening interventions. Individuals could also consider trying to treat themselves as long as their healing methods did not infringe upon the rights of others. Finally, [like] architects and . . . all other professionals, uncertified practitioners could not say they are certified. (Ullman, 1981)

This completely *laissez-faire* approach is not likely to materialize in the near future. Allopathy will still insist on restrictive licensing laws, especially in areas that pertain to services normally provided by physicians. On the other hand, alternative practices will become legitimized in regions where alternative practitioners and their clients exert local political pressure. This has already been demonstrated by the pro-laetrile lobby, by acupuncture and by chiropractic.

Establishing Regulation and Standards of Practice

The attitude of organized medicine, which maintains that it will control alternative healing and oppose the government-sponsored regulation of such healing as an independent entity, is not in the interest of public health. Most professions, especially new ones, need public funding to start professional societies, prepare certifying examinations, establish independent certifying commissions and monitor standards of practice. Money should also be made available for public and professional education, for establishing fair procedures for the review of negligence or impaired practice and for participation in the legislative process. Both the new physician assistant and nurse practitioner programs received liberal federal funding and money from private foundations for these purposes during the early 1970's. However, virtually no money has been made available to the new alternative healing professions for this purpose.

Without regulatory control, individual practitioners work in isolation, and there is little public accountability for questions of negligence, malpractice or impaired practice due to alcohol or drug abuse. When the responsibility for control rests with the individual consumer, there may be no effective means of pursuing grievances. Furthermore, legal actions initiated by consumers are extremely costly and time consuming, and judgments may not be obtainable when practitioners leave to work in another state. Moreover, this type of regulation does not prevent negligence from occurring *before* it harms the client. Because of all these factors, leaving regulation solely in the hands of the consumer puts an unfair burden on the alternative health-care client who, because of illness or psychological stress, may be severely hampered in his or her ability to fully pursue a grievance.

Some observers, like Jerry Green, hope that a method of regulation can be adopted that allows the alternative professions to grow and be judged by their own standards. In an article that appeared in *Wholistic Dimensions in Healing* he set out his goal:

> Our current legal structure does not purport to comprehend health practices outside the medical model. Nor does it

> intend to prohibit them. [The] system was designed to offer preservation for standards of training and practice in medicine. Can they be applied to new perspectives on health that evolve outside of the medical model?
>
> The wholistic professions should be given time to articulate their own standards of training and practice. New laws will be necessary to establish procedures regulating licensure and competency in practice. Our choice lies between measuring new horizons by yesterday's concepts and developing a new conceptual framework to suit our experiences of today. (Kaslof, 1978)

Before the new healing disciplines can develop their own standards of practice, they will have to develop strong professional organizations that can address the questions raised by Jerry Green. Unfortunately, this may not be easy in some of these disciplines. Many of the new practitioners are extremely individualistic in their philosophy and lifestyle, and resent professional control of any form. As yet only chiropractic has been successful in molding a nationally cohesive professional society. But if there is a backlash leveled at the new practices from the ranks of allopathy, such strong professional societies will be needed to fight the challenge of orthodoxy.

Clearly, a fair method of regulation is needed for the new healing professions. This is in the best interests of both the consumer and the alternative healing disciplines. The system should emphasize the quality of care and accountability to the public, as well as allowing the new professions a chance to elaborate standards that meet the future needs of their own disciplines. In other words, regulation should not hamper the growth of the new healing professions, but should foster high standards for safety, honesty and professional accountability.

chapter 9

The Future of the New Medicine

The future of alternative healing is as uncertain as its meteoric rise. Fads in healing, as in other disciplines, are easily spread via the media and advertising. It is far more difficult to establish healing practices that have long-term durability.

The Cost of Health Care

Health care continues to be a major financial burden on both the individual and society, accounting for almost 10% of the entire gross national product. Health-care costs continue to rise faster than the rate of inflation, and the bulk of health-care dollars provide services for the minority of people who require institutional care.

During the 1970's alternative medicine began to address these issues. Some conventional health-care analysts looked to the new medicine as a way of reducing costs through preventing disease. A few corporations encouraged health practices on the job that included exercise, stress reduction, nutritional planning and counseling. Walter J. McNerney, then President of the Illinois Blue Cross Association, spoke for the need to promote cost effective health practices along holistic lines:

> Probably the most significant sign that the wholistic fires are going to spread rather than languish is the [great support it is getting] from industry and third-party payers. As a third-party payer, let me be the first here to say without hesitation that our interest in the wholistic concept does not arise solely from an impassioned concern for the quality of life of our millions of subscribers and their families. The money that Blue Cross Plans and insurance companies are spending on preventive services, health education and health improvement programs for their subscribers, policy holders, employees and communities . . . flows instead from our concern [over] the explosion of health care costs. (Cunningham, 1977)

But the alternative healing practices have yet to document cost effectiveness in the areas of disease prevention. Moreover, the alternative healers have not defined their role in preventive care. Conventional medicine has chosen to focus on discovering illness in its early stages. This includes screening for cervical cancer with the Pap smear, recording blood pressure to uncover hypertension, routine blood and urine tests for diabetes and sampling the stool for blood to detect early intestinal cancer. This view has been criticized by some as locking the barn door after the horse has left; but alternative healing has provided no well-thought-out system for well-being.

The view of the new medicine on prevention remains extremely simple in its scope. One study, performed by Dr. Lester Breslow, dean of UCLA's School of Public Health, found that seven health practices recommended by many new healers correlated with increased longevity. They were: getting regular exercise, not smoking, maintaining normal weight, eating breakfast, avoiding the heavy use of alcohol, sleeping about 8 hours each night and eschewing snacks between meals. But while few public health experts would disagree with these recommendations, they do not form a comprehensive public health policy.

A pilot project utilizing pastoral counseling in conjunction with holistic health care was begun in a free clinic in Springfield, Ohio and later expanded to suburban Chicago. The program was sponsored by the Department of Preventive Medicine and Community Health of the University of Illinois School of Medicine. The goals of the project were summarized as follows:

> Patient education programs [must] emphasize the wholistic rather than the partistic nature of personal health, and . . . encourage the development of healthy lifestyles that will prevent the onset of illness. Great emphasis on education should, in the long run, prove to be more economical than our present crisis care (reactive) system.

The theory of this activity is sensible, but as yet unproven. We do not know if holism is applicable to the general population. The suburban Chicago aspect of the project, where the test group is predominantly middle to upper income, and comprises a medically sophisticated population, may not reflect the impact of health teaching on poor rural or urban sectors of society, or in already medically underserved areas.

Another factor in the economy of alternative healing is that insurance carriers do not generally reimburse for client counseling, biofeedback training or relaxation instruction, for example, and the few that do reimburse do so at a rate far lower than they do for standard medical services. If third-party payers would increase their reimbursement of alternative services to rates equivalent to those for allopathic medical services, the cost of the new medicine might equal or exceed the cost of the current system. In the Utah study already cited, patients treated by chiropractors and allopaths had similar costs associated with their care. Thus we cannot predict whether holistic practices will in reality lower health-care costs.

Individual Responsibility for Health

Alternative healing has been criticized for narrowly focusing the responsibility for health on the individual. Rick Carlson, a California attorney and proponent of alternative medicine, explained the role of the individual in health practices at a 1975 Conference on Future Directions in Health Care sponsored by the Rockefeller Foundation:

> The assumption is not made in holistic thinking—as it is in modern medicine—that health is the product of specific interventions into the body and biochemistry of the patient. Rather, the concept of holism as applied to medical care presumes that health for both the individual and the population can be achieved only by intervention on many

> levels of human experience . . . that the individual can be healthy only if the physical environment and the social and cultural dimensions of life are conducive to health. Superimposed on this model is the recognition of the importance of and the need for individual assumption of responsibility for health.

In recent years this view has been labeled as "blaming the victim." Critics of this view state that most cancers, for example, may be environmentally produced through pollution of the air, water and land, and from occupational hazards, rather than being due to some fault of the individual. Similarly it is hard to blame the residents of communities where toxic wastes have been dumped, or soldiers who have been exposed to radiation or agent orange while in the military, for the harmful effects of these substances. Poverty, racism and sexism are all known to contribute to disease. Poor and nonwhite people have higher-than-average death rates, including unusually high death rates due to accidents, homicide, suicide, alcohol and drug abuse.

It is doubtful whether any form of medicine can make significant inroads into the overall health of the population without addressing the evils of modern industrial and urban living. And this requires organized group effort, not isolated individual action.

Therapeutic Efficacy

All forms of medical therapy are potentially beneficial because of the placebo effect. This does not make the cure or relief any less real, but it does point to the nonspecific nature of each therapy. The new healers stress a more humanistic client-therapist interaction that can be expected to catalyze the placebo effect. The positive publicity that surrounds many of the new healing practices further enhances the faith of the client.

This enhancement of the placebo effect is one of the major contributions of alternative medicine. Through its criticism of the technological depersonalization of medical care and its reintroduction of the human element to the healing setting, it may have made a profound contribution to the healing arts. Yet it is questionable to license and institutionalize practices that rely solely on placebo effects; there is a difference between the faith healing at Lourdes and the medical services offered by acupuncturists, chiropractors, herbalists and other alternative healers. Because of this, new healers must prove the effectiveness of their specific methods. They may not choose to do it in the allopathic model, but they owe the consumer some test of the therapeutic effectiveness of their methods.

Unfortunately, there is little evidence with which to substantiate the use of many of the new therapies. Biofeedback and relaxation have begun to amass a body of information that helps in analyzing their effectiveness and appropriate use in the treatment of illness. They have been shown to have applicability in the area of stress-related illness, such as hypertension; and possibly—along with psychological counseling—in the treatment of anxiety-related problems. Specific neurological disorders such as fecal incontinence or paralysis that results from spinal cord injury or stroke may also be amenable to biofeedback training. However, we do not yet know whether meditation, biofeedback, relaxation or autogenic training will promote a high level of well-being or prevent stress-related disease.

Nor do we yet know their effectiveness in treating diseases of the internal organs.

Acupuncture is just beginning to test its effectiveness in the Western model of clinical trials. The use of acupuncture for surgical anesthesia has been disappointing despite the fact that early reports indicated its widespread applicability in this area. Similarly, the effectiveness of the traditional use of acupuncture to balance body energy or treat organ dysfunction remains to be proven.

Chiropractic is particularly interesting in that it is a treatment that has grown in popularity despite a paucity of evidence to support its effectiveness and has survived in the face of continued attack from conventional medicine. The chiropractic claim of being "a portal of entry" into the health care system shocks the majority of allopaths, yet chiropractors appear to have a growing following in the general public. However, we still do not know why and how chiropractic manipulation works, or whether spinal manipulation is an effective treatment for such diverse medical problems as heart ailments, gynecological disorders and emotional illness.

Similarly, little is known about the effectiveness of the alternative drug therapies. Homeopathy is perplexing in that its remedies are often so diluted that no chemical evidence of their presence can be detected by standard assay techniques.

It is also difficult to understand why so many people believe in vitamins and other "natural" remedies. Perhaps it is because they are available without a prescription, and the public is eager to control its own health care. Thus, while self-diagnosis and self-medication are anathema to many physicians, they are indications that a segment of the population wants control over its own bodies. However, the effectiveness of these substances in either treating or preventing all but rare illnesses has never been documented. Moreover, they can be poisonous. Until proven otherwise, their use will remain a large-scale placebo experiment.

The growth of alternative healing continues to be paradoxical. On the one hand modern society appears to be wed to technological discovery; most people look to bioscience as the foundation of medical care, even though there is ample information to support the notion that medicine has only a minimal effect on good health and longevity. At the same time a growing segment of the population is rejecting scientific medicine in favor of alternative practices that have humanistic and religious appeal, despite the fact that they have not been proven useful by rigorous scientific standards.

Legal Regulation

Errors in allopathic care, even uncommon ones, are both expensive and tragic. A study of surgical errors at a major teaching hospital revealed that 36 cases of mismanagement cost over $1 million. Twenty of the 36 patients died as a result of surgical error, and 5 of the 16 survivors left the hospital with major permanent injury.

Errors in purely medical care are probably even more common. A study at a Boston teaching center showed that 36% of the patients suffered an iatrogenic illness (illness caused by medical care) during their hospital stay. Over 40% of the affected patients had between 2 and 7 adverse reactions to their therapy, and 5% of the patients died as a result. The authors of the study concluded that the risk of untoward reactions among hospitalized patients was greater than the risk of heart attack in the general population. (Steel, 638)

No similar information exists for patients who use alternative therapies. If there are dangers related to these new treatments, we do not yet know how great they are. However, at least some risks—a few of which have been described in this book—are associated with these therapies, and some form of regulation is needed to insure that the public is protected from impaired, incompetent or negligent practitioners.

The alternative healers argue that they should not be regulated by the allopathic healing industry. They say that the economic incentives are so great that allopathy is unlikely to regulate them fairly. There seems to be substance to their argument. It is not in the self-interest of allopathic practitioners—who receive about one-quarter of the $200 billion yearly income of allopathic medicine in the United States—to admit competition from alternative healers. Moreover, allopathic medicine has a long history of waging propaganda campaigns against competitive healers. Regulatory bodies dominated by conventional physicians are likely to control the alternative healing industry for their own benefit. This may not always be in the public's best interest, and is not likely to promote the growth of the new healing disciplines. Professional societies can elaborate their own standards for training and practice, but the new healers have been slow to form the necessary organizations.

Thus, some fair method of regulation must be formulated that allows consumers the freedom to choose the type of health care they wish while at the same time protecting them from unscrupulous and dangerous practitioners. To date, alternative health care remains largely unregulated, and a truly fair system has not been formulated.

Moreover, if the political and economic climate favors government retreat from the role of providing the funding that new professions need for establishing training programs, providing certifying examinations, and monitoring practice, the new healers may find it extremely difficult to establish the necessary framework with which to control and direct their burgeoning professions.

Most observers point out the obvious: that some of the new therapies will fade from favor, some will become incorporated into conventional medicine and others will remain independent healing professions. However, it is extremely difficult to predict which healing arts will fall into each category. Proven therapeutic effectiveness may not be the basis upon which the public chooses which alternative practices will remain and which will ultimately fall by the wayside.

Bibliography

Agras, W., et al. Relaxation training. *Archives of General Psychiatry,* Vol. 37, pp. 859–863, 1980.

Albany Medical College. *Medical History and Physical Examination.* Albany, NY: Albany Medical College, 1973.

American Chiropractic Association. *Chiropractic: State of the Art.* Des Moines, IA: American Chiropractic Association, 1981.

American Holistic Medical Association. *Newsletter,* p. 1, November, 1978.

American Medical Association. *Proceedings of the Third National Congress on Medical Quackery.* Chicago: American Medical Association, 1961.

American Psychiatric Association. Task force on vitamin therapy in psychiatry. *Nutrition Review, Suppl.,* Vol. 44, pp. 44–47, July, 1974.

Anderson, T. Large-scale trials of vitamin C. *Annals of the New York Academy of Sciences,* Vol. 258, pp. 498–504, 1975.

Arcamone, F., and Cassinelli, G. New antitumor drugs from plants. *Journal of Ethnopharmacology,* Vol. 2, pp. 149–160, 1980.

Arnold, L., et al. Megavitamins for minimal brain dysfunction: a placebo-controlled study. *Journal of the American Medical Association*, Vol. 240, No. 24, pp. 2642–2643, 1978.

Australia Committee of Inquiry into Chiropractic, Osteopathy, Homeopathy and Naturopathy. *Report.* Canberra: Australia Government Publishing Service, 1977.

Ayman, D. An evaluation of therapeutic results in essential hypertension. *Journal of the American Medical Association,* Vol. 95, No. 4, pp. 246–249, 1930.

Barrett, S., and Knight, G. *The Health Robbers.* Philadelphia: George Stickley, 1976.

Barton, C. Placebo analgesia. *Western Journal of Medicine,* Vol. 132, No. 5, p. 474, 1980.

Basmajian, J. *Biofeedback: Principles and Practice for Clinicians.* Baltimore: Williams and Wilkins, 1979.

Beatty, J., and Legewie, H. (eds). *Biofeedback and Behavior.* New York: Plenum Press, 1976.

Beecher, H. Surgery as a placebo effect. *Journal of the American Medical Association,* Vol. 176, No. 13, pp. 1102–1107, 1961.

Benson, H. Angina pectoris and the placebo effect. *New England Journal of Medicine,* Vol. 300, No. 5, pp. 1424–1429, 1979.

Benson, H. *The Mind/Body Effect.* New York: Simon and Schuster, 1979.

Benson, H. Systemic hypertension and the relaxation response. *New England Journal of Medicine,* Vol. 296, No. 20, pp. 1152–1155, 1977.

Benson, H. and Epstein, H. The placebo effect: a neglected asset in the care of patients. *Journal of the American Medical Association,* Vol. 232, No. 12, pp. 1225–1227, 1975.

Benson, H., et al. Decreased blood pressure in borderline hypertensive subjects who practiced meditation. *Journal of Chronic Diseases,* Vol. 27, pp. 163–169, 1974.

Benson, H., et al. Decreased blood pressure in pharmacologically treated hypertensive patients who regularly elicited the relaxation response. *Lancet,* Vol. 1, No. 7852, pp. 289–291, 1974.

Berkeley Holistic Health Center. *The Holistic Health Handbook.* Berkeley, CA: And/Or Press, 1978.

Berliner, H., and Salmon, J. The holistic alternative to scientific medicine: history and analysis. *International Journal of Health Services,* Vol. 10, No. 1, pp. 133–147, 1980.

Bin, Hsu. The use of herbs as anticancer agents. *American Journal of Chinese Medicine*, Vol. 3, No. 4, pp. 301–306, 1980.

Blackwell, B., et al. Transcendental meditation in hypertension. *Lancet,* Vol. 1, No. 7953, pp. 223–226, 1976.

Blaine, E. Manipulative (chiropractic) dislocations of the atlas. *Journal of the American Medical Association*, Vol. 85, pp. 1356–1359, 1925.

Blanchard, B. Effect of music on pulse rate, blood pressure and final exam scores of university students. *Journal of School Health*, Vol. 49, No. 8, pp. 470–471, 1979.

Bonica, J. Therapeutic acupuncture in the people's republic of china. *Journal of the American Medical Association,* Vol. 228, No. 12, pp. 1544–1551, 1974.

Bourdillon, J. *Spinal Manipulation.* New York: Appleton-Century-Crofts, 1973.

Boyd, H. Homeopathic medicine [letter]. *British Journal of Medicine,* Vol. 1, No. 6166, pp. 821–822, 1979.

Bresler, D., and Kroenig, R. A three-factor theory of acupuncture. Paper presented for Acupuncture Research Project.

Los Angeles, University of California, Los Angeles School of Medicine, 1975.

Brooks, P. Chinese herbal arthritis cure and agranulocytosis. *Medical Journal of Australia,* Vol. 2, pp. 860, 1977.

Broussard, R. Using relaxation for COPD. *American Journal of Nursing,* Vol. 11, pp. 1962–1963, 1979.

Buerger, A., and Tobis, J. *Approaches to the Validation of Manipulation Therapy.* Springfield, IL: Charles C. Thomas, 1975.

Bunker, J., and Gerber, W. Holistic health care and California's Board of Medical Quality Assurance. *Western Journal of Medicine,* Vol. 131, No. 6, pp. 480–484, 1979.

Callan, J. Holistic health or holistic hoax. *Journal of the American Medical Association,* Vol. 241, No. 11, pp. 1156, 1979.

Caper, P. Competition and health care. *New England Journal of Medicine,* Vol. 304, No. 21, pp. 1296–1298, 1981.

Carlson, R. *The End of Medicine.* New York: John Wiley & Sons, 1975.

Carlson, R. Holism and reductionism as perspectives in medicine and patient care. *Western Journal of Medicine,* Vol. 131, No. 6, pp. 466–470, 1979.

Carr-Kaffashan, L., and Woolfolk, R. Active and placebo effects in treatment of moderate and severe insomnia. *Journal of Consulting and Clinical Psychology,* Vol. 47, No. 6, pp. 1072–1080, 1979.

Cashman, L. Herbal medicines and rheumatoid arthritis [letter]. *British Medical Journal,* Vol. 2, No. 6168, p. 504, 1979.

Cassileth, B., et al. Information and participation preferences among cancer patients. *Annals of Internal Medicine,* Vol. 92, No. 6, pp. 832–836, 1980.

Centers for Disease Control. Poisoning associated with herbal teas. *Morbidity and Mortality Weekly Reports.* Vol. 26, No. 32, 1977.

Chan, H. Lead poisoning from ingestion of Chinese herbal medicine. *Clinical Toxicology,* Vol. 10, No. 3, pp. 273–281, 1977.

Chapman, L., et al. Evoked potential assessment of acupunctural analgesia: attempted reversal with naloxone. *Pain,* Vol. 9, No. 2, pp. 183–197, 1980.

Chung, S. Pain, enkephalin and acupuncture. *Nature,* Vol. 283, No. 5744, pp. 243–244, 1980.

Coan, R. The acupuncture treatment of low back pain: a randomized controlled study. *American Journal of Chinese Medicine,* Vol. 8, Nos. 1–2, pp. 181–189, 1980.

Cochrane, A. *Effectiveness and Efficacy in Health Services.* London: Nuffield Provincial Hospitals Trust, 1971.

Cohen, H. Regulatory politics and American medicine. *American Journal of Behavioral Science,* Vol. 19, pp. 122–136, 1975.

Cohen, H.D., et al. A double-blind methodology for biofeedback research. *Psychophysiology,* Vol. 14, pp. 603–608, 1977.

Comroe, J. The witch doctor, the which doctor and the wish doctor. *American Review of Respiratory Diseases,* Vol. 120, pp. 1189–1195, 1979.

Cooper, M., et al. A relaxation technique in the management of hypercholesteremia. *Journal of Human Stress,* Vol. 5, No. 4, pp. 24–27, 1979.

Costilo, L. Competition policy and the medical profession. *NewEnglandJournalofMedicine,* Vol. 304, No. 8, p. 1099, 1981.

Cott, A. Megavitamins: the orthomolecular approach to behavioral disorders and learning disabilities. *Academic Therapeutics,* Vol. 7, pp. 245–258, 1972.

Coulter, H. *Divided Legacy-A History of the Schism in Medical Thought.* Vols. 1,2,3. Washington, D.C.: Weehawken Book Co., 1977.

Coulter, H. Homeopathy and modern medical science. *Journal of the American Institute of Homeopathy.* Vol. 73, No. 3, 1980.

Cousins, N. A layman looks at truth telling. *Journal of the American Medical Association,* Vol. 244, No. 17, pp. 1929–1930, 1980.

Cousins, N. *Anatomy of an Illness as Perceived by the Patient.* New York: W.W. Norton, 1979.

Cox, D., et al. Differential effectiveness of EMG feedback, verbal relaxation instruction and medication placebo with tension headache. *Journal of Consulting and Clinical Psychology,* Vol. 43, pp. 892–898, 1975.

Cranton, E. Letter to author. February 24, 1981.

Creagan, R., et al. Failure of high dose vitamin C therapy to benefit patients with advanced cancer: a controlled trial. *New England Journal of Medicine,* Vol. 301, No. 13, pp. 687–690, 1979.

Crelin, E. A scientific test of the chiropractic theory. *American Scientist,* Vol. 61, pp. 574–580, 1973.

Culliton, B., and Waterfall, W. Chiropractors and the AMA. *British Medical Journal,* Vol. 1, No. 6161, p. 467, 1979.

Cunningham, R., and Westberg, J. (eds). *Report of National Symposium on Wholistic Health Care.* Oak Brook, IL: W.K. Kellogg Foundation, 1977.

Curran, W. Acupuncture: The practice of medicine and the right to demand medical services. *New England Journal of Medicine,* Vol. 305, No. 8, pp. 439–440, 1981.

Curran, W. Reasonableness and randomization in clinical trials: fundamental law and government regulation. *New England Journal of Medicine,* Vol. 300, No. 22, pp. 1273–1275, 1979.

Davis, W. Competition in health care. *New England Journal of Medicine,* Vol. 304, No. 20, p. 1240, 1981.

Desai, I., et al. A clinical study of infective hepatitis treated with liv-52. *Indian Pediatr,* Vol. 14, No. 3, pp. 197–202, 1977.

Dollery, C. A bleak outlook for placebos (and for science). *European Journal of Clinical Pharmacology,* Vol. 15, pp. 219–221, 1979.

Doran, D., and Newell, D. Manipulation in treatment of low back pain. *British Journal of Medicine,* Vol. 2, pp. 161–165, 1975.

Duhl, L. The social context of health. In Hastings, A., et al. (eds): *Health and the Whole Person.* Boulder, CO: Westview Press, 1980, p. 43.

Dunea, G. Healing by touching. *British Journal of Medicine,* Vol. 1, No. 6165, pp. 795–796, 1979.

Editorial. The flight from science. *British Medical Journal,* Vol. 280, No. 6026, pp. 1–3, 1980.

Editorial. Deaths from coffee enemas. *Journal of the American Medical Association,* Vol. 244, No. 14, pp. 1608–1610, 1980.

Editorial. High tea. *Medical Journal of Australia,* Vol. 2, No. 5, p. 232, 1979.

Elliott, H. The clinical pharmacology of a herbal asthma cigarette. *British Journal of Clinical Pharmacology,* Vol. 10, No. 5, pp. 487–490, 1980.

Engel, G. The clinical application of the biophysical model. *American Journal of Psychiatry,* Vol. 137, No. 5, pp. 535–544, 1980.

Engel, G. The need for a new medical model. *Science,* Vol. 196, No. 4286, pp. 129–136, 1977.

Feldenkrais, M. *The Case of Nora.* New York: Harper and Row, 1977.

Fielding, J., et al. A program for prevention in Massachusetts. *Preventive Medicine,* Vol. 7, pp. 564–640, 1978.

Findley, T. The omnipresent placebo effect [letter]. *New England Journal of Medicine,* Vol. 301, No. 11, p. 614, 1979.

Fink, D. Holistic health implications for health planning. *American Journal of Health Planning,* Vol. 1, pp. 12–20, 1976.

Folb, P. *The Safety of Medicines.* Berlin: Springer-Vorlag, 1980.

Fong, T. Problems associated with megadose vitamin C therapy. *Western Journal of Medicine,* Vol. 134, No. 3, p. 264, 1981.

Ford, F., and Clark, D. Thrombosis of the basilar artery with softening of the cerebellum and brain stem due to manipulation of the neck. *Bulletin of the Johns Hopkins Hospital,* Vol. 98, pp. 37–42, 1956.

Fox, C. The Feldenkrais phenomenon. Reprinted from *Quest/80,* December–January, 1978.

Fox, E., and Melzack, R. Transcutaneous electrical stimulation and acupuncture. Comparison for treatment of low back pain. *Pain,* Vol. 2, No. 2, p. 146, 1976.

Frank, J. *Persuasion and Healing.* Baltimore: Johns Hopkins University Press, 1972, p. 47.

Gable, M. Medical self-sufficiency. *San Francisco Magazine,* pp. 42–43, January, 1980.

Gatchel, R., and Price, K. *Clinical Applications of Biofeedback: Appraisal and Status.* New York: Pergamon Press, 1979.

Gates, G. Thomsonian medicine and early georgian medical societies. *Journal of the Medical Association of Georgia,* Vol. 66, No. 1, pp. 23–27, 1977.

Gibson, R. Homeopathic therapy in rheumatoid arthritis: evaluation by double-blind clinical trial. *British Journal of Clinical Pharmacology,* Vol. 9, No. 5, pp. 453–459, 1980.

Gibson, R., et al. Salicylates and homeopathy in rheumatoid arthritis: preliminary observations. *British Journal of Clinical Pharmacology,* Vol. 6, No. 5, pp. 391–395, 1978.

Golden, G. Nonstandard therapies in the developmental disabilities. *American Journal of the Diseases of Childhood,* Vol. 134, No. 5, pp. 487–491, 1980.

Goldman, B., et al. Effects of zen meditation on anxiety reduction and perceptual functioning. *Journal of Consulting and Clinical Psychology,* Vol. 47, No. 3, pp. 551–557, 1979.

Goldring, W., et al. Reassurance in the management of benign hypertensive disease. *Circulation,* Vol. 14, pp. 260–265, 1956.

Green, J. Contracts with your doctor? *New Realities,* Vol. 2, No. 1, 1978.

Green, J. New roles for changing times. In Kaslof, L. (ed): *Wholistic Dimensions in Healing: A Resource Guide.* New York: Doubleday-Dolphin, 1978. Provided by author.

Green, J. Responsibility for health. 1976. Provided by author.

Green, J., and Markell, S. The health care contract: a model for sharing responsibility. *Holistic Health Review,* Vol. 4, No. 1, pp. 18–28, 1981. Reprint provided by author.

Greenberg, D. The case against laetrile: the fraudulent cancer remedy. *Cancer,* Vol. 45, No. 4, pp. 799–808, 1980.

Guirdham, A. *The Nature of Healing.* London: George Allen and Unwin, Ltd., 1964.

Gunn, C. Dry needling of muscle motor points for chronic low back pain: a randomized clinical trial with long term follow up. *Spine,* Vol. 5, No. 3, pp. 279–291, 1980.

Haldeman, S., and Drum, D. The compression subluxation. *Journal of Clinical Chiropractic Archives Education,* Vol. 1, p. 10, 1971.

Haldeman, S. *Modern Developments in the Principles and Practice of Chiropractic.* New York: Appleton-Century-Crofts, 1979.

Hanus, S., et al. Vertebral artery occlusion complicating yoga exercises. *Archives of Neurology,* Vol. 34, pp. 574–575, 1977.

Harris, D. Editorial. *Journal of Holistic Health,* Vol. 5, pp. 1–2, 1980.

Harvard Medical School. How to evaluate medical information. *Harvard Medical School Health Letter,* Vol. 3, No. 7, p. 6, 1978.

Harvey, J., et al. Mistletoe hepatitis. *British Medical Journal,* Vol. 8, No. 6259, pp. 186–187, 1981.

Hasselberg, P. *Report of the Commission of Inquiry into Chiropractic in New Zealand.* Wellington, New Zealand: Government Printer, 1979.

Healthview Newsletter. Interview with Dr. William Kelley. Vol. 1, No. 4, pp. 1–11, 1977.

Heintz, G., et al. Why are naturopathic preparations purchased in health food stores? *Lakartidningan,* Vol. 75, No. 35, pp. 2951–2953, 1978.

Hellerstein, D. Cures that kill. *Harper's Magazine,* pp. 20–24, December, 1980.

Herbert, V. Facts and fictions about megavitamin therapy. *Resident and Staff Physician,* Vol. 24, pp. 43–50, 1978.

Herbert, V. Laetrile: The cult of cyanide. Promoting poison for profit. *American Journal of Clinical Nutrition,* Vol. 32, pp. 1121–1158, 1979.

Herbert, V. Letter. *American Journal of Clinical Nutrition,* Vol. 33, No. 1, p. 10, 1980.

Herbert, V. Megavitamin therapy. *Journal of the American Pharmacological Association,* Vol. 17, pp. 764–766, 1977.

Herbert, V. Pangamic acid ("Vitamin B15"). *American Journal of Clinical Nutrition,* Vol. 32, pp. 1534–1540, 1979.

Herbert, V. The vitamin craze. *Archives of Internal Medicine,* Vol. 140, No. 2, pp. 173–176, 1980.

Hindmarsh, K., and LeGatt, D. Mexican drug therapy. *Clinical Toxicology,* Vol. 17, pp. 85–99, 1980.

Hiroria, I. Carcinogenic activity of *symphytum officinale. Journal of the National Cancer Institute,* Vol. 61, No. 3, pp. 865–869, 1978.

Hitokoto, H., et al. Fungal contamination and mycotoxic detection of powdered herbal drugs. *Applied Environmental Microbiology,* Vol. 36, No. 2, pp. 252–256, 1978.

Hoffer, A., and Osmond, H. Schizophrenia: a new approach. *Journal of Mental Science,* Vol. 100, pp. 29–45, 1954.

Howe, G. *Cure or Heal?* London: George Allen and Unwin, Ltd., 1965.

Hunt, V., et al. *A Study of Structural Integration from Neuromuscular Energy, Field and Emotional Approaches.* Boulder, CO: Rolf Institute, 1977.

Huxtable, R. Herbal teas and toxins. Novel aspects of pyrrolizidine poisoning in the United States. *Perspectives in Biology and Medicine,* Vol. 24, No. 1, pp. 1–14, 1980.

Hyder, A. Letter to the author. October 16, 1981.

Inglis, B. *The Case for Unorthodox Medicine.* New York: G.P. Putnam's Sons, 1965.

Jaffe, D. *Healing from Within.* New York: Alfred A. Knopf, 1980.

Kapadia, G., et al. Carcinogicity of *camella sinensis* (tea) and some tanin-containing folk medicinal herbs administered subcutaneously in rats. *Journal of the National Cancer Institute,* Vol. 57, No. 1, pp. 207–209, 1976.

Kaslof, L. (ed). *Wholistic Dimensions in Healing: A Resource Guide.* New York: Doubleday-Dolphin, 1978.

Kay, R. Zinc and copper in human nutrition. *Journal of Human Nutrition,* Vol. 35, pp. 25–36, 1981.

Kirkendall, W. Danger of megavitamin therapy [letter]. *Journal of the American Medical Association,* Vol. 239, No. 25, p. 2658, 1978.

Knowles, J. Conference: Future Directions in Health Care, December 10–11, 1975. Sponsored by the Rockefeller Foundation, New York.

Knowles, J. *Doing Better and Feeling Worse.* New York: W.W. Norton, 1977.

Knox, V., et al. Subject expectancy and the reduction of cold pressor pain with acupuncture and placebo analgesia. *Psychosomatic Medicine,* Vol. 41, No. 6, pp. 477–483, 1979.

Krieger, D. Therapeutic touch and healing energies from laying on of hands. *Journal of Holistic Health,* Vol. 1, p. 24, 1976.

Kubista, E., et al. Electro-acupuncture's influence on the closure mechanism of the female urethra in incontinence. *American Journal of Chinese Medicine,* Vol. 4, No. 2, pp. 177–181, 1976.

Lamontagne, Y., et al. Acupuncture for smokers: lack of long-term therapeutic effect in a controlled study. *Canadian Medical Association Journal,* Vol. 122, No. 7, pp. 787–790, 1980.

Lange, R. Holistic medicine. Is all holistic medicine whole? *New York State Journal of Medicine,* Vol. 80, No. 6, pp. 996–999, 1980.

Leonard, G. The holistic health revolution. *New West Magazine,* pp. 40–49, May 10, 1976.

Leonard, G. The holistic health revolution. *Journal of Holistic Health,* Vol. 2, p. 80, 1977.

Leonard, G. Sociological implications of holistic health. *Journal of Holistic Health,* Vol. 3, p. 11, 1978.

Leung, P. Treatment of low back pain with acupuncture. *American Journal of Chinese Medicine,* Vol. 7, No. 4, pp. 372–378, 1979.

Levine, J., et al. The mechanism of placebo analgesia. *Lancet,* Vol. 2, No. 8091, pp. 654–657, 1978.

Lieberman, L., et al. O'leary and bourkovic's conceptualization of placebo: the placebo paradox. *American Psychologist,* Vol. 34, No. 6, pp. 553–554, 1979.

Lief, R., et al. (eds). *The Psychological Basis of Medical Practice.* New York: Harper and Row, 1963, p. 167.

Lightfoote, J., et al. Lead intoxification in an adult by Chinese herbal medication. *Journal of the American Medical Association,* Vol. 238, No. 14, p. 1539, 1977.

Loomis, E. The correlation of medicine and religion, a holistic approach. *Journal of Holistic Health,* Vol. 1, pp. 56–70, 1976.

Lowenthal, M., et al. Aplastic anemia and optic fundus hemorrhages due to traditional herbal remedies. *Journal of Tropical Medicine and Hygiene,* Vol. 81, No. 9, pp. 177–179, 1978.

Malizia, E., et al. Electroacupuncture and peripheral beta endorphin and ACTH levels [letter]. *Lancet,* Vol. 2, No. 8141, pp. 535–536, 1979.

Marini-Bettolo, G. Present aspects of the use of plants in traditional medicine. *Journal of Ethnopharmacology,* Vol. 2, pp. 5–7, 1980.

Marwick, C. Religion and medicine draw closer. *Medical World News,* Vol. 19, pp. 26–33, December 25, 1978.

McGarey, W. Applying edgar cayce readings to the daily clinical practice of medicine. *Journal of Holistic Medicine,* p. 1, September, 1976.

Meares, A. What can the cancer patient expect from intensive meditation. *Australian Family Physician,* Vol. 9, pp. 322–325, 1980.

Medical Letter. Toxic reactions to plant substances sold in health food stores. *Med Letter,* Vol 21, No. 7 Issue 528, April 6, 1979.

Mendelsohn, G., et al. Acupuncture anesthesia for low back pain. *Clinical and Experimental Neurology,* Vol. 15, pp. 182–185, 1978.

Mendelsohn, R. I no longer believe in modern medicine. *The New Physician,* pp. 18–26, 1980.

Miller, N. Biofeedback: Evaluation of a new technique. *New England Journal of Medicine,* Vol. 290, No. 12, pp. 876–879, 1974.

Mills, D. *Royal Commission on Health Services Study of Chiropractors, Osteopaths and Naturopaths in Canada.* Ottawa: Queen's Printer and Controller of Stationery, 1966.

Mould, R. Clinical trial design in cancer. *Clinical Radiology,* Vol. 30, pp. 371–381, 1979.

National Nutrition Consortium. *Report of the Committee on Safety, Toxicity and Misuse of Vitamins and Trace Minerals.* Chicago: American Dietetic Association, 1978.

Nelson, R. Are clinical trials pseudoscience? *Forum on Medicine,* pp. 594–600, 1979.

Newton, G., et al. Amygdalin toxicity studies in rats predict chronic cyanide poisoning in humans. *Western Journal of Medicine,* Vol. 134, pp. 97–103, 1981.

Nuechterlein, K., and Holroyd, G. Biofeedback in the treatment of tension headache. *Archives of General Psychiatry,* Vol. 37, pp. 867–873, 1980.

Oleson, T. An experimental evaluation of auricular diagnosis. The somatic mapping of musculoskeletal pain at ear acupuncture points. *Pain,* Vol. 8, No. 2, pp. 217–219, 1980.

Osler, W. *The Principles and Practice of Medicine.* New York: D. Appleton, 1909.

Otto, H., and Kinight, J. *Dimensions in Wholistic Healing.* Chicago: Nelson-Hall, 1979.

Parker, G., and Tupling, H. The chiropractic patient: psychosocial aspects. *Medical Journal of Australia,* Vol. 2, No. 10, pp. 373–378, 1976.

Parker, G., and Tupling, H. Consumer evaluation of natural therapies and general practitioners. *Medical Journal of Australia,* Vol. 1, No. 17, pp. 619–622, 1977.

Parker, G., et al. A controlled trial of cervical manipulation for migraine. *Australia-New Zealand Medical Journal,* Vol. 8, pp. 589–593, 1978.

Parker, G., et al. New Zealand inquiry into chiropractic. *Medical Journal of Australia,* Vol. 1, No. 3, pp. 103–105, 1980.

Parker, G., et al. Why does migraine improve during a clinical trial? Further results from a trial of cervical manipulation for migraine. *Australia-New Zealand Medical Journal,* Vol. 10, pp. 192–198, 1980.

Parkin, P., et al. Vertebral artery occlusion following manipulation of the neck. *New Zealand Medical Journal,* Vol. 88, No. 625, pp. 441–443, 1979.

Parsons, J. Contaminated herbal tea as a potential source of arsenic poisoning. *North Carolina Medical Journal,* Vol. 42, No. 1, pp. 38–39, 1981.

Patel, C. Biofeedback-aided relaxation and meditation in the management of hypertension. *Biofeedback and Self Regulation,* Vol. 2, pp. 1–41, 1977.

Patel, C. Randomized control trial of yoga and biofeedback in management of hypertension. *Lancet,* Vol. 2, No. 7925, pp. 93–95, 1975.

Patel, C. Twelve month follow up of yoga and biofeedback in the management of hypertension. *Lancet,* Vol. 1, No. 7898, pp. 62–64, 1975.

Patel, C. Yoga and biofeedback in the management of hypertension. *Lancet,* Vol. 2, No. 7837, pp. 1053–1055, 1973.

Pauling, L. Orthomolecular psychiatry. *Science,* Vol. 160, pp. 265–271, 1968.

Peek, C. A critical look at the theory of placebo. *Biofeedback and Self Regulation,* Vol. 2, No. 4, pp. 325–335, 1977.

Pelletier, K. *Holistic Medicine.* New York: Delacorte Press, 1979.

Pelletier, K. Holistic medicine from pathology to prevention. *Western Journal of Medicine,* Vol. 131, pp. 481–484, 1979.

Pelletier, K. *Mind as Healer, Mind as Slayer. A Holistic Approach to Preventing Stress Disorders.* New York: Delacorte and Delta, 1977.

Pellettiri, L. Introduction. *Journal of Holistic Health,* Vol. 1, p. 1, 1976.

Petkov, V. Plants with hypotensive, antiatheromatous and coronary dilating action. *American Journal of Chinese Medicine,* Vol. 3, No. 3, pp. 197–236, 1979.

Picci, V. The exploitation of medicinal plants of the mediterranean area. *Journal of Ethnopharmacology,* Vol. 2, pp. 81–89, 1980.

Pierce, R. *The Rolfing Technique of Connective Tissue Manipulation.* Boulder, CO: Rolf Institute, 1976.

Pomerantz, B., and Cheng, R. Suppression of noxious responses in single neurons of cat spinal cord by electroacupuncture and its reversal by the opitate antagonist naloxone. *Experimental Neurology,* Vol. 64, pp. 327–341, 1979.

Pomerantz, B., and Paley, D. Electroacupuncture hypalgesia is mediated by afferent nerve impulses: an electrophysiological study in mice. *Experimental Neurology,* Vol. 66, pp. 398–401, 1979.

Pratt-Thomas, H., and Beyer, K. Cerebellar and spinal injuries after chiropractic manipulation. *Journal of the American Medical Association,* Vol. 133, pp. 600–603, 1947.

Relman, A. Chiropractic: recognized but unproved [editorial]. *New England Journal of Medicine,* Vol. 301, No. 12, pp. 659–660, 1979.

Relman, A. The ethics of randomized clinical trials: two perspectives. *New England Journal of Medicine,* Vol. 300, No. 22, p. 1272, 1979.

Reuler, J., et al. The chronic pain syndrome: misconceptions and mismanagement. *Annals of Internal Medicine,* Vol. 93, pp. 588–596, 1980.

Rich, W. Acupuncture for arthritis [letter]. *Medical Journal of Australia,* Vol. 2, No. 6, pp. 311–312, 1979.

Rich, J., and Sloan, R. A relaxation technique. *American Journal of Nursing,* Vol. 80, No. 11, pp. 1960–1964, 1979.

Ries, C., and Sahud, M. Agranulocytosis caused by chinese herbal medicines. *Journal of the American Medical Association,* Vol. 231, p. 352, 1975.

Roberts, H. Dolomite as a source of toxic metals. *New England Journal of Medicine,* Vol. 54, No. 7, p. 423, 1981.

Rolf, I. Structure—a new factor in understanding the human condition. Presented June 10, 1978, at the Explorers of Humankind Conference. Boulder, CO: Rolf Institute, 1978.

Rolf, I. Structural integration. *Confining Psychiatrica,* Vol. 16, pp. 69–79, 1973.

Rosenberg, L. Vitamin dependent genetic disease. *Hospital Practice,* Vol. 5, No. 7, pp. 59–66, 1970.

Roth, J. *Health Purifiers and Their Enemies.* New York: Prodist, 1977.

Rywerant, Y. Improving the ability to perform. *Somatics,* Vol. 1, No. 2, pp. 37–39, 1977.

Rywerant, Y. The story of hanoch's return to the flute. *Somatics,* Vol. 2, No. 3, pp. 26–29, 1979.

Sadr, A., et al. Granulomatose peritonitis due to *sofia. International Surgeon,* Vol. 62, Nos. 6–7, pp. 364–365, 1977.

Sainani, G. Onion, garlic and experimental atherosclerosis. *Japanese Heart Journal,* Vol. 20, No. 3, pp. 351–357, 1979.

Sayed, M. Traditional medicine in health care. *Journal of Ethnopharmacology,* Vol. 2, pp. 19–22, 1980.

Scarf, M. Images that heal. *Psychology Today,* pp. 33–46, 1980.

Schaefer, R. *Chiropractic: State of the Art.* Des Moines, IA: American Chiropractic Association, 1979.

Schapiro, A. A contribution to the history of the placebo effect. *Behavioral Science,* Vol. 5, pp. 109–135, 1960.

Schapiro, A. Factors contributing to the placebo effect. *American Journal of Psychotherapy,* Vol. 18, Suppl. 1, pp. 73–88, 1964.

Schapiro, A. The placebo effect in the history of medical treatment: implications for psychiatry. *American Journal of Psychiatry,* Vol. 116, pp. 298–304, 1959.

Schindel, L. Placebos: a review. *Israel Medical Journal,* Vol. 18, pp. 275–280, 1959.

Schneider, D. *Revolution in the Body/Mind.* East Hampton, NY: Alexa Press, 1977.

Schoemaker, J., and Tasto, D. The effects of muscle relaxation on blood pressure of essential hypertension. *Behavioral Research Therapy,* Vol. 13, pp. 29–43, 1975.

Schwartz, G., et al. Posterior inferior cerebral artery syndrome of Wallenberg after chiropractic manipulation. *Archives of Internal Medicine,* Vol. 97, p. 352, 1956.

Seer, P. Psychological control of essential hypertension: a review of the literature and methodological critique. *Psychological Bulletin,* Vol. 86, No. 5, pp. 1015–1043, 1979.

Shapiro, A. The reliability and validity of a placebo test. *Journal of Psychiatric Research,* Vol. 15, No. 4, pp. 253–290, 1979.

Shapiro, J., and Shapiro, D. The psychology of responsibility: some second thoughts on holistic medicine. *New England Journal of Medicine,* Vol. 301, No. 4, pp. 211–212, 1979.

Shapiro, S., and Lerner, D. Psychophysiological effects of autogenic training and progressive relaxation. *Biofeedback and Self Regulation,* Vol. 5, No. 2, p. 249, 1980.

Simon, A., et al. An evaluation of iridology. *Journal of the American Medical Association,* Vol. 242, No. 13, pp. 1385–1389, 1979.

Simonton, O., and Mathews-Simonton, S. *Getting Well Again.* Los Angeles: J.P. Tarcher, 1978.

Sjolund, B., and Erikson, M. Electro-acupuncture and endogenous morphines. *Lancet,* Vol. 2, No. 7994, p. 1085, 1976.

Sjolund, B., et al. The influence of naloxone on analgesia produced by peripheral conditioning stimulation. *Brain Research,* Vol. 173, No. 2, pp. 295–301, 1979.

Smith, R. *At Your Own Risk: The Case Against Chiropractic.* New York: Trident Press, 1969.

Smits, H. The PSRO in perspective. *New England Journal of Medicine,* Vol. 305, No. 5, pp. 253–258, 1981.

Sodipo, J. Therapeutic acupuncture for chronic pain. *Pain,* Vol. 7, No. 3, pp. 359–365, 1979.

Soprano, K. *The Utilization of Chiropractic in Central Massachusetts.* Worcester, MA: The College of the Holy Cross, 1974.

Stanford Research Institute. *Chiropractic in California.* Los Angeles: The Hayes Foundation, 1960.

Stang, J., and Stang, O. Religion and medicine at the crossroads: (w)holistic health care. *Ohio State Medical Journal,* Vol. 75, No. 12, pp. 769–772, 1979.

Steel, K., et al. Iatrogenic illness on a general medical service at a university hospital. *New England Journal of Medicine,* Vol. 304, No. 11, pp. 638–642, 1981.

Stegar, J., et al. Comprehensive biofeedback versus self monitored relaxation in the treatment of tension headache. *Headache,* Vol. 20, No. 3, pp. 137–142, 1980.

Stephenson, J. Homeopathic philosophy in the light of twentieth century physics. *Journal of the American Institute of Homeopathy,* p. 67, 1960.

Stone, R., and DeLeo, J. Psychotherapeutic control of hypertension. *New England Journal of Medicine,* Vol. 294, No. 2, pp. 80–84, 1976.

Svihus, R. On healing the whole person: a perspective. *Western Journal of Medicine,* Vol. 131, No. 6, pp. 478–480, 1979.

Svihus, R. Origins and definitions. *Journal of Holistic Health,* Vol. 2, pp. 17–22, 1977.

Task Force Report. *Megavitamins and Orthomolecular Therapy in Psychiatry.* Washington, D.C.: American Psychiatric Association, 1973.

Taub, E. Integrative medicine. *Journal of Holistic Health,* Vol. 5, pp. 77–85, 1980.

Taylor, C., et al. Relaxation therapy and high blood pressure. *Archives of General Psychiatry,* Vol. 34, pp. 339–432, 1977.

Thompson, T. Chiropractic [letter]. *New England Journal of Medicine,* Vol. 302, No. 6, pp. 354, 1980.

Thomson, W. *Herbs That Heal.* New York: Charles Scribner's Sons, 1976.

Todd, M. Forward. *Journal of Holistic Health,* Vol. 2, p. 1, 1975.

Travel, J., and Rinzler, R. The myofascial genesis of pain. *Postgraduate Medicine,* Vol. 11, p. 425, 1952.

Tsuei, J., et al. Influence of acupuncture stimulation during pregnancy: the induction and inhibition of labor. *Obstetrics and Gynecology,* Vol. 50, No. 4, pp. 479–488, 1977.

Tubesing, R., et al. The wholistic health center project: an action research model for providing preventive, whole-person health care at the primary level. *Medical Care,* Vol. 15, No. 3, pp. 217–227, 1977.

Ullman, D. Getting beyond medical chauvinism. Unpublished paper supplied to the author by Mr. Ullman, 1981.

Ullman, D. Holistic health as a model for personal and social change. *Journal of Alternative Human Services,* pp. 9–12, 1979.

Ullman, D. Implications of a court case. In *Holistic Health Handbook.* Berkeley Holistic Health Center, Berkeley, CA: And /Or Press, 1978.

Ullman, D. Responsibility and holistic health. Holistic health news. Paper supplied to the author by Mr. Ullman, 1980.

Underwood, E. Trace metals in human and animal health. *Journal of Human Nutrition,* Vol. 35, No. 1, pp. 37–48, 1981.

Vitler, R. Nutritional aspects of ascorbic acid: uses and abuses. *Western Journal of Medicine,* Vol. 133, No. 6, pp. 485–492, 1980.

Vogel, A., et al. The therapeutics of placebo. *American Family Physician,* Vol. 21, No. 7, pp. 105–109, 1980.

Waddell, D. "Alternative" medicine in a county hospital clinic. In: Environments for Humanized Health Care. Symposium sponsored by the University of California, Berkeley, March 8, 1979.

Wallace, D. Thomsonians: the people's doctors. *Clio Medica,* Vol. 3, No. 4, pp. 169–186, 1980.

Wallace, R. Physiological effects of transcendental meditation. *Science,* Vol. 167, p. 1751, 1970.

Wallis, R., and Morley, P. (eds). *Marginal Medicine.* New York: Free Press, 1976.

Wardwell, W. Sounding board. *New England Journal of Medicine,* Vol. 302, No. 12, pp. 688–690, 1980.

Watts, M. (ed). Orthodox medicine, humanistic medicine, holistic health care. *Western Journal of Medicine,* Vol. 131, No. 6, p. 463, 1979.

West, M. Meditation. *British Journal of Psychiatry,* Vol. 135, pp. 457–467, 1979.

Wickramaseka, I. A conditioned response model of the placebo effect: predictions from the model. *Biofeedback and Self Regulation,* Vol. 5, No. 1, pp. 5–18, 1980.

Wittenborn, J., et al. Niacin in the long-term treatment of schizophrenia. *Archives of General Psychiatry,* Vol. 28, p. 308, 1973.

Wolf, S. Effects of suggestion and conditioning on the action of chemical agents in human subjects: the pharmacology of placebos. *Journal of Clinical Investigation,* Vol. 29, pp. 100–109, 1950.

Wolfe, S. *Pills That Don't Work.* New York: Farrar, Straus & Giroux, 1980.

Woolley, F., and Kane, R. A comparison of allopathic and chiropractic care. In Buerger, A., and Tobis, J. (eds): *Approaches to the Validation of Manipulative Therapy.* Springfield, IL: Charles C. Thomas, 1977.

Yahn, G. The impact of holistic medical groups and health concepts. *Journal of the American Medical Association,* Vol. 242, No. 20, pp. 2202–2205, 1979.

Young, J. *The Medical Messiahs. A Social History of Health Quackery in 20th Century America.* Princeton, NJ: Princeton University Press, 1967.

Young, V. Nutrients, vitamins and minerals in cancer prevention: facts and fallacies. *Cancer,* Vol. 43, pp. 2125–2136, 1979.

Young, W. Herbal enema, colitis and stricture. *British Journal of Radiology,* Vol. 53, No. 627, pp. 248–249, 1980.

Zellen, M. A new design for randomized clinical trials. *New England Journal of Medicine,* Vol. 300, No. 22, pp. 1242–1245, 1979.

Index